Getting Ready for My Eye Surgery

Eye Surgery Book for Kids – Preparation and Recovery

This book belongs to:

Written by Dr. Fei Zheng-Ward   Illustrated by Moch. Fajar Shobaru

Copyright © 2025 Fei Zheng-Ward

All rights reserved. Published by Fei Zheng-Ward, an imprint of FZWbooks. No part of this book may be copied, reproduced, recorded, transmitted, or stored by any means or in any form, electronic or mechanical, without obtaining prior written permission from the copyright owner.

Identifiers: ISBN 979-8-89318-077-0 (eBook)
                      ISBN 979-8-89318-078-7 (paperback)
                      ISBN 979-8-89318-079-4 (hardcover)

Did you notice that people have different eye colors?

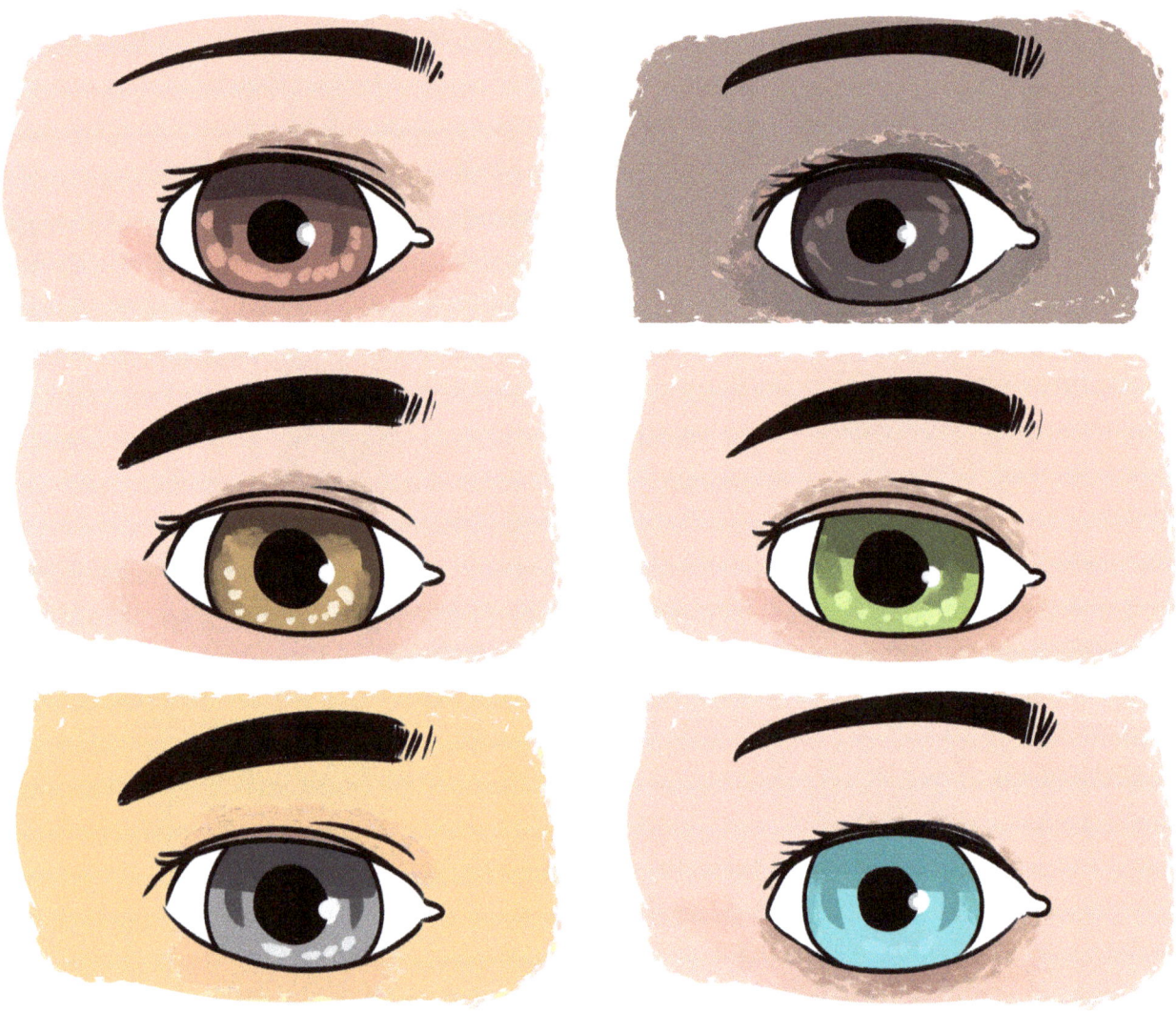

What color(s) are your eyes?

Circle your answer(s) below.

Brown   Hazel   Blue   Amber   Gray   Green   Other

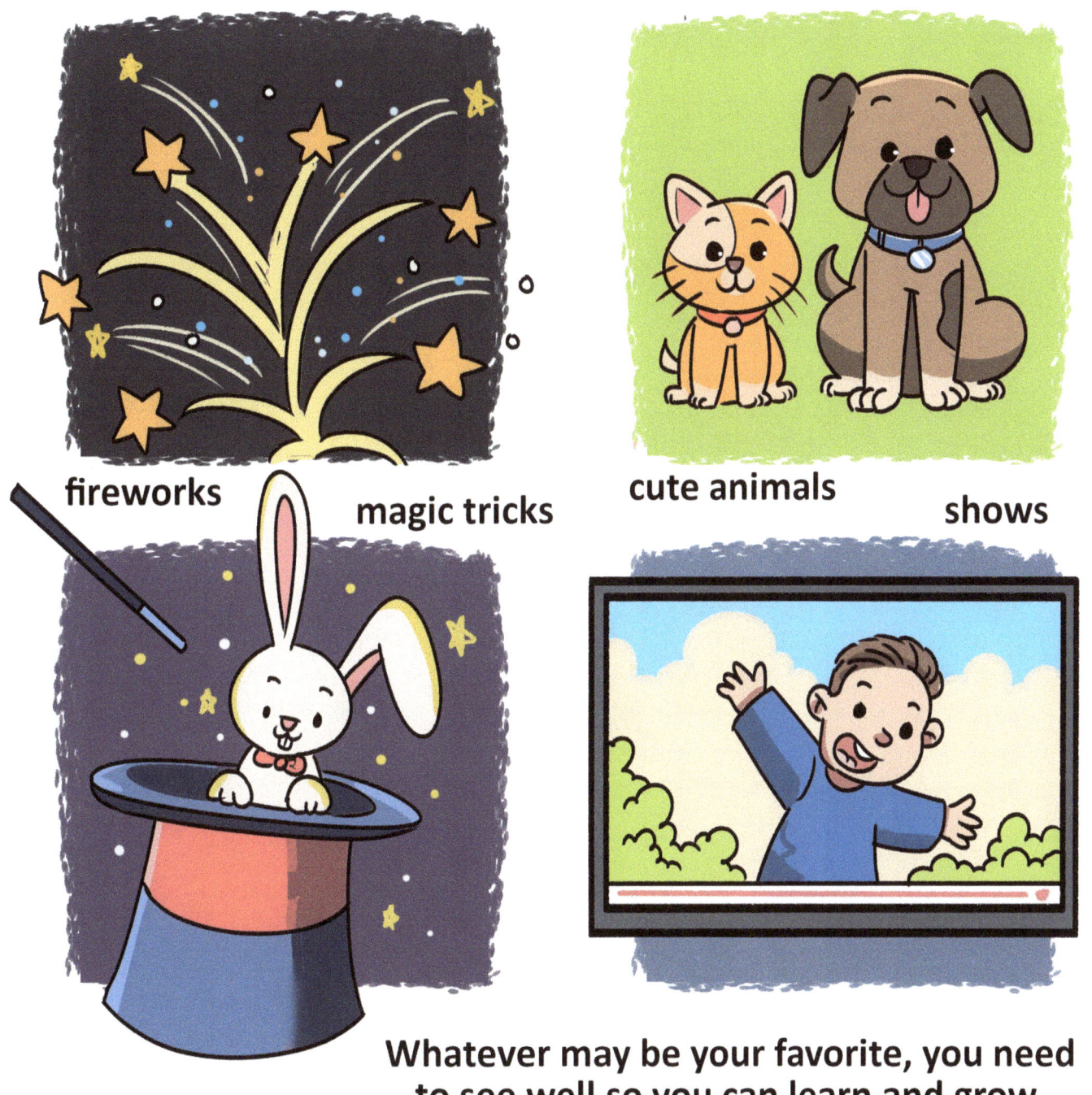

Each eye has different parts.

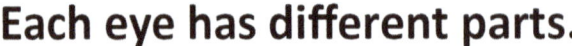

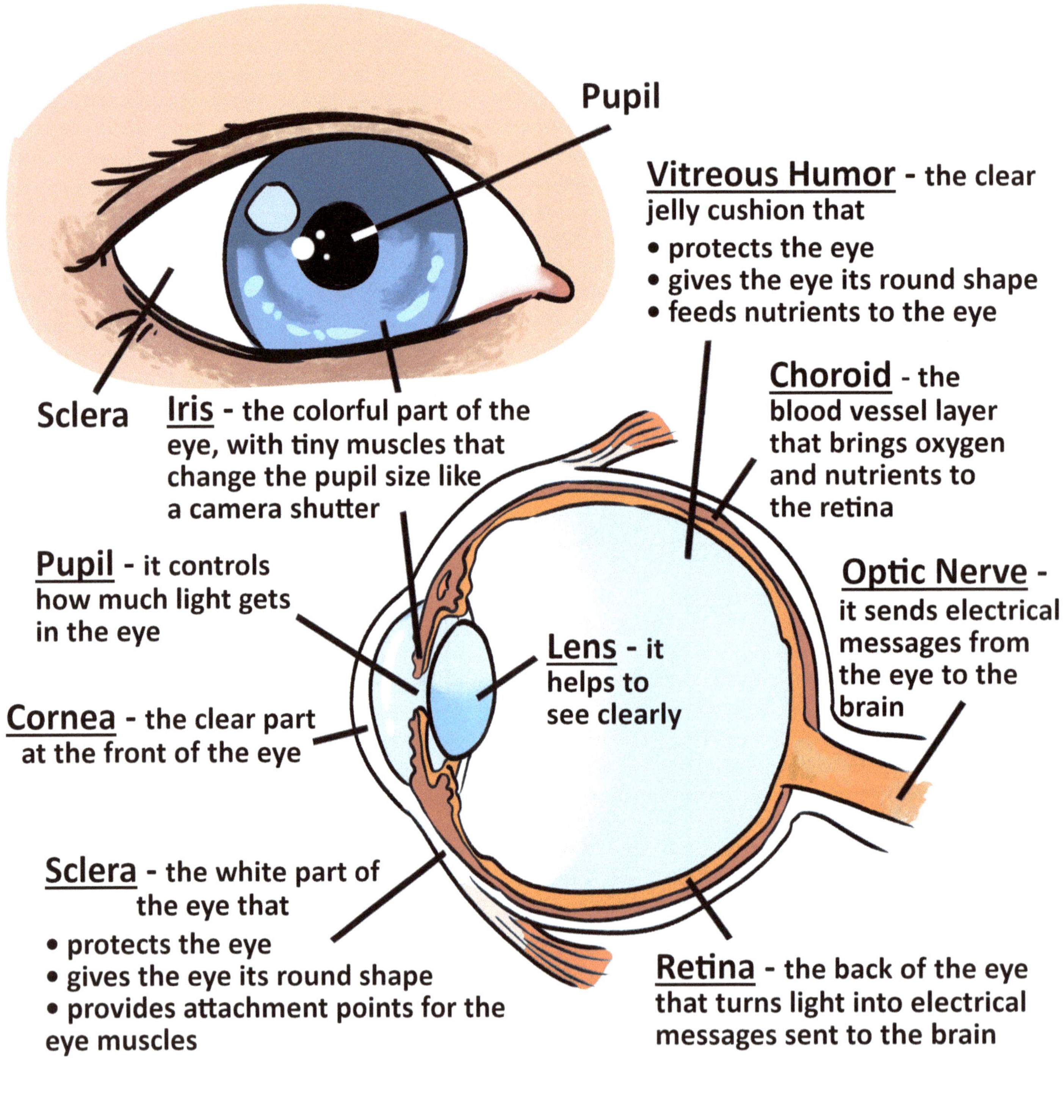

Pupil

Vitreous Humor - the clear jelly cushion that
- protects the eye
- gives the eye its round shape
- feeds nutrients to the eye

Sclera

Iris - the colorful part of the eye, with tiny muscles that change the pupil size like a camera shutter

Choroid - the blood vessel layer that brings oxygen and nutrients to the retina

Pupil - it controls how much light gets in the eye

Lens - it helps to see clearly

Optic Nerve - it sends electrical messages from the eye to the brain

Cornea - the clear part at the front of the eye

Sclera - the white part of the eye that
- protects the eye
- gives the eye its round shape
- provides attachment points for the eye muscles

Retina - the back of the eye that turns light into electrical messages sent to the brain

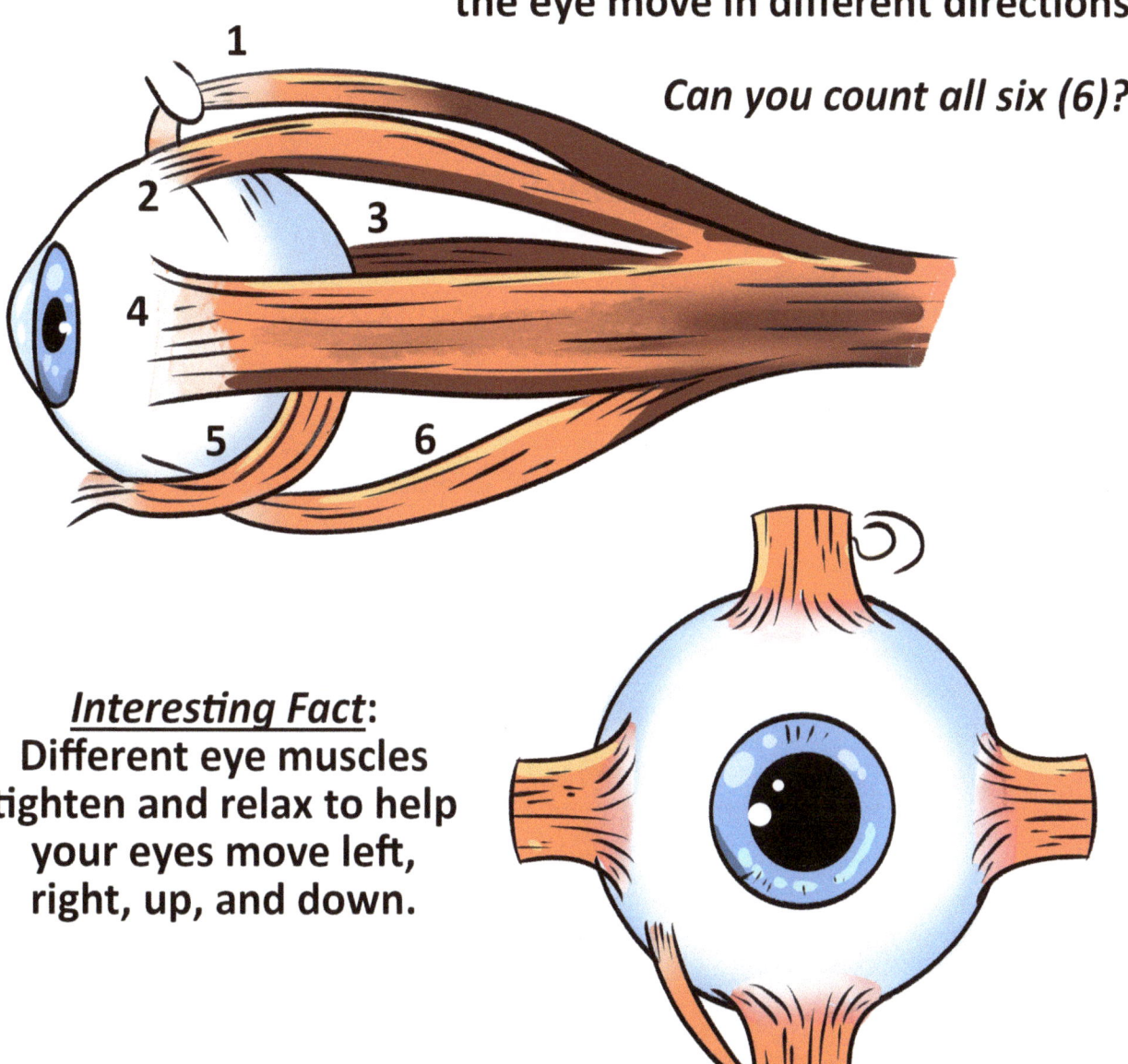

There are six (6) different muscles that control each eye, and they help the eye move in different directions.

Can you count all six (6)?

Interesting Fact: Different eye muscles tighten and relax to help your eyes move left, right, up, and down.

Here's how your eye works:

Light enters through your **cornea** and passes through the **pupil** to reach the **lens**.

The **lens** focuses the light on the **retina**.

The **retina** turns the light into electrical messages that get delivered through the **optic nerve** to your **brain**.

Your brain then tells you what you're seeing.

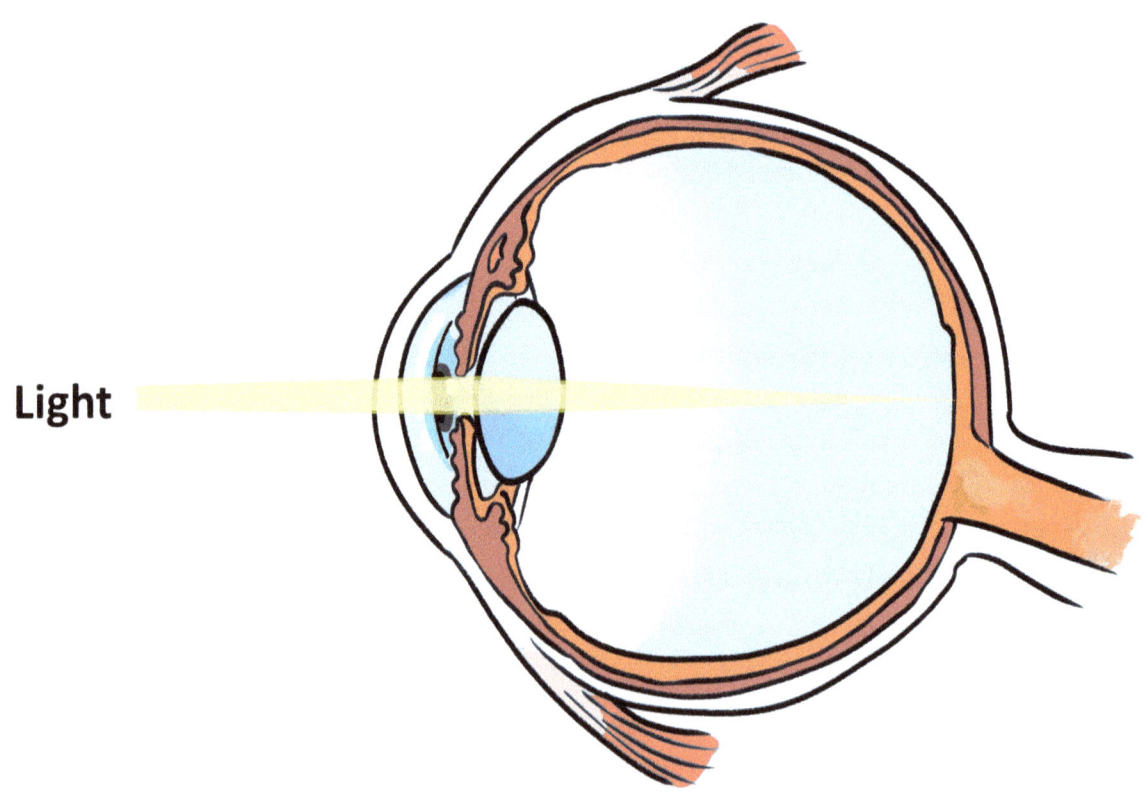

Light

LIGHT → CORNEA → PUPIL → LENS

↓

BRAIN ← OPTIC NERVE ← RETINA

<u>Fun fact</u>: Did you know your retina sees things upside-down, and your brain makes them right-side up?

Cool, right?

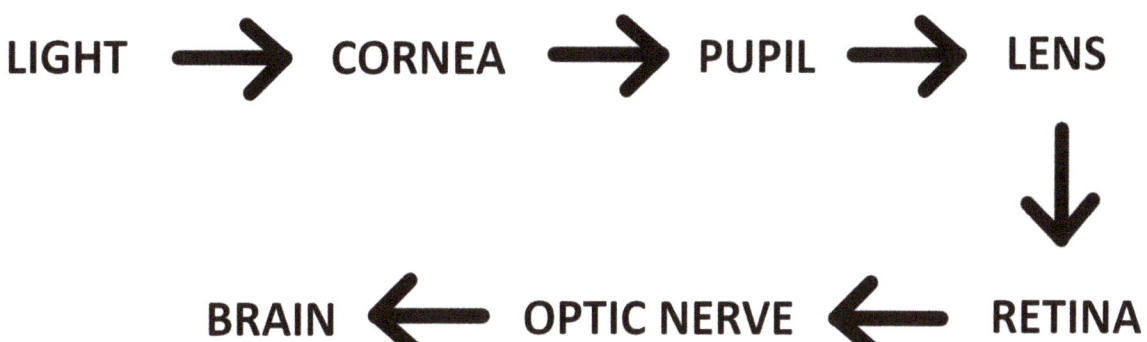

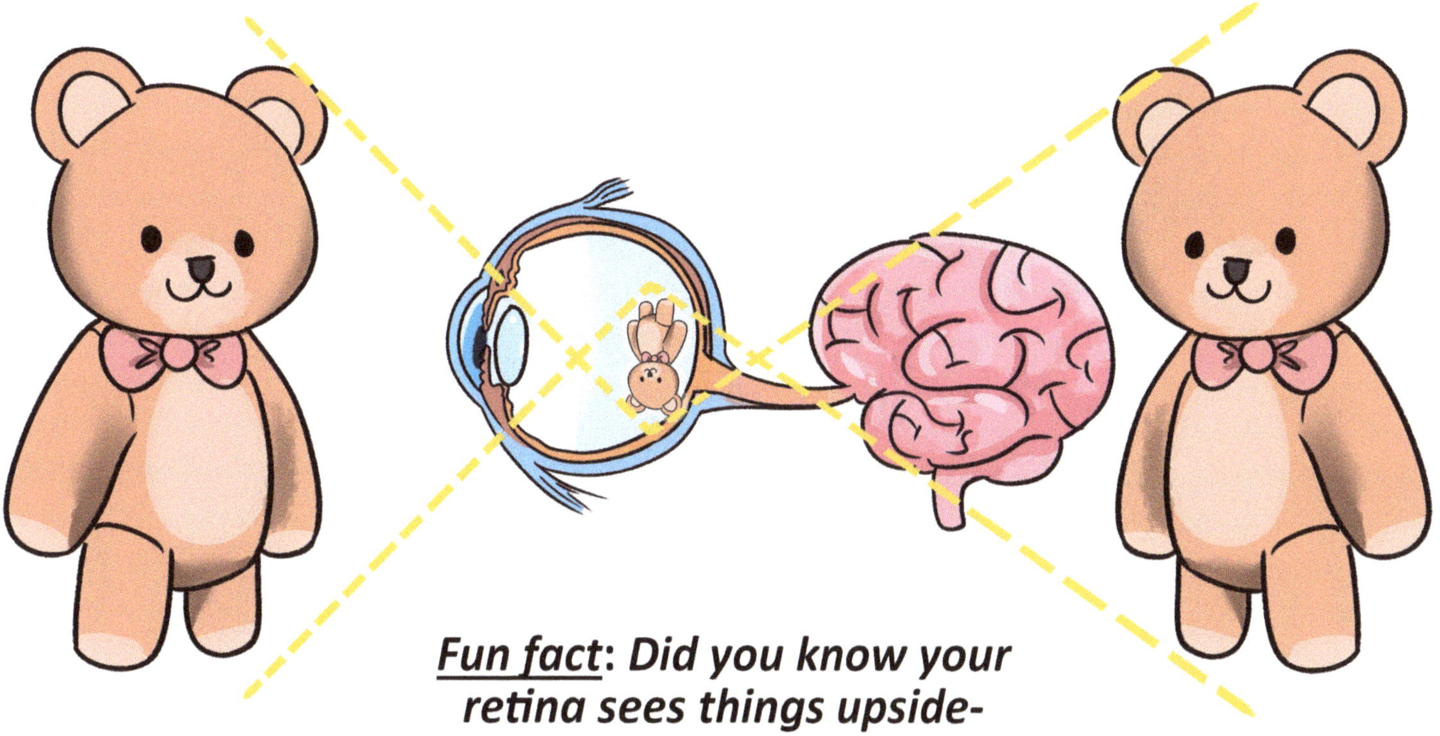

For children, one of the most common eye surgeries is to repair the eye muscles.

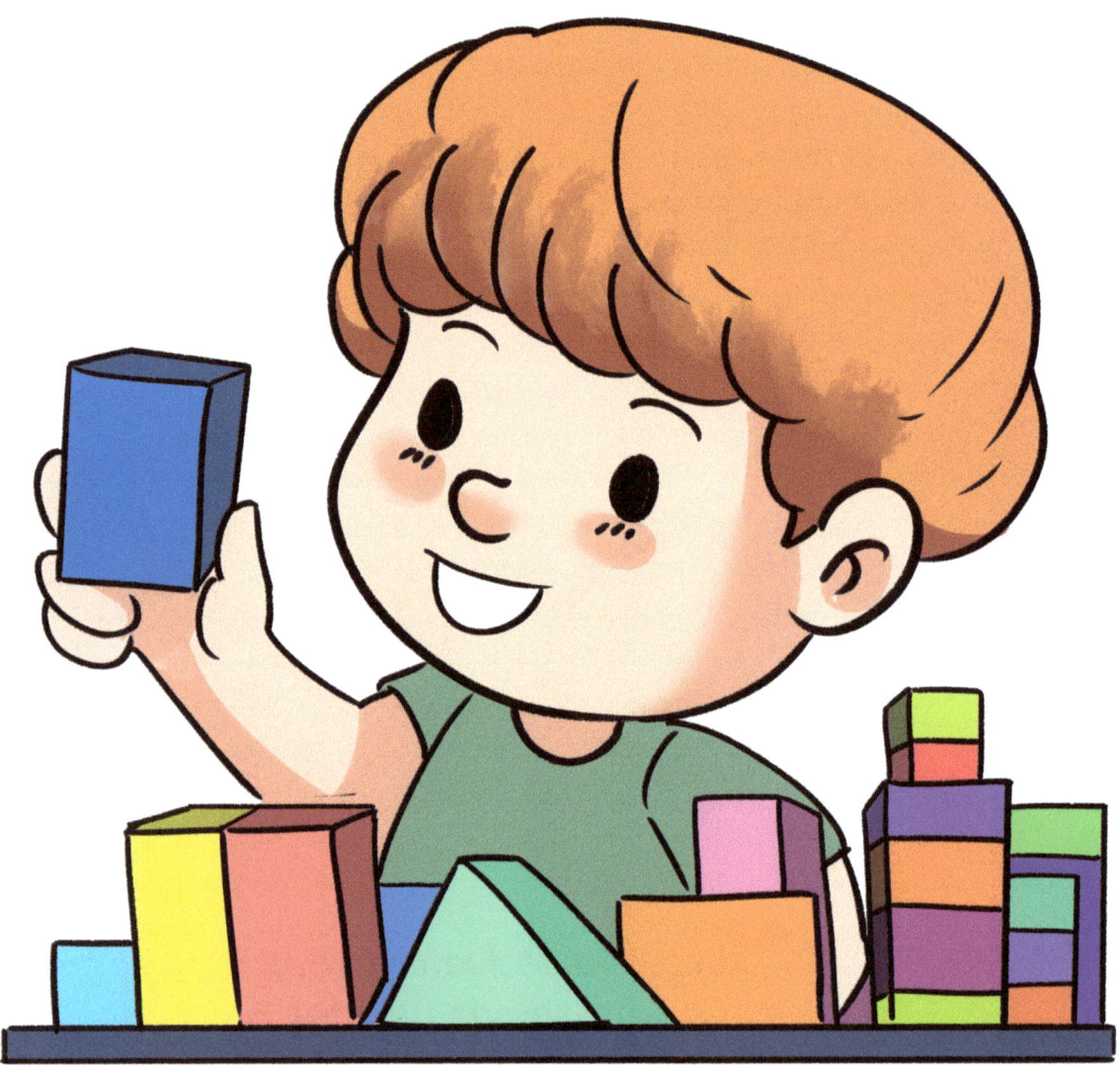

When your eye muscles work well together, they help your eyes see exactly where things are so you can reach out and grab them easily.

If your eye muscles are too tight or too loose, your eyes might see two puppies instead of one. This is called double vision, and it confuses your brain.

Over time, your brain blocks out the electrical messages from the weaker eye.

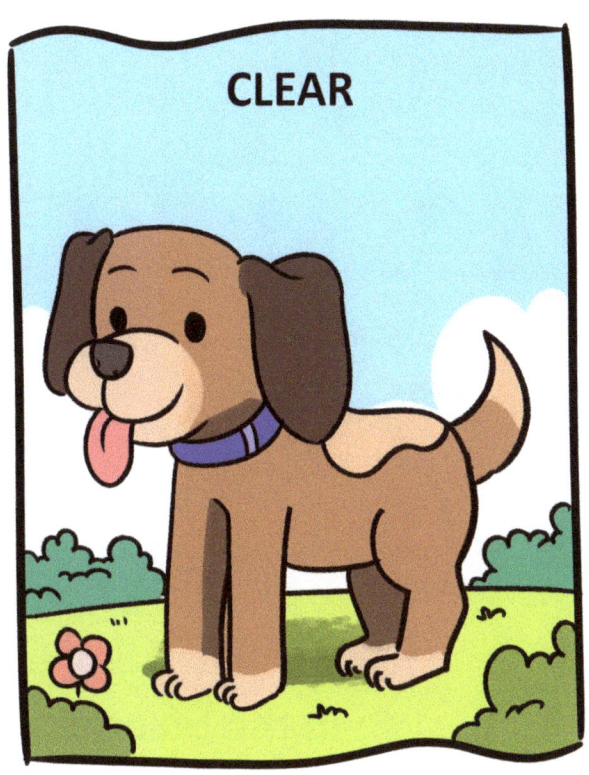
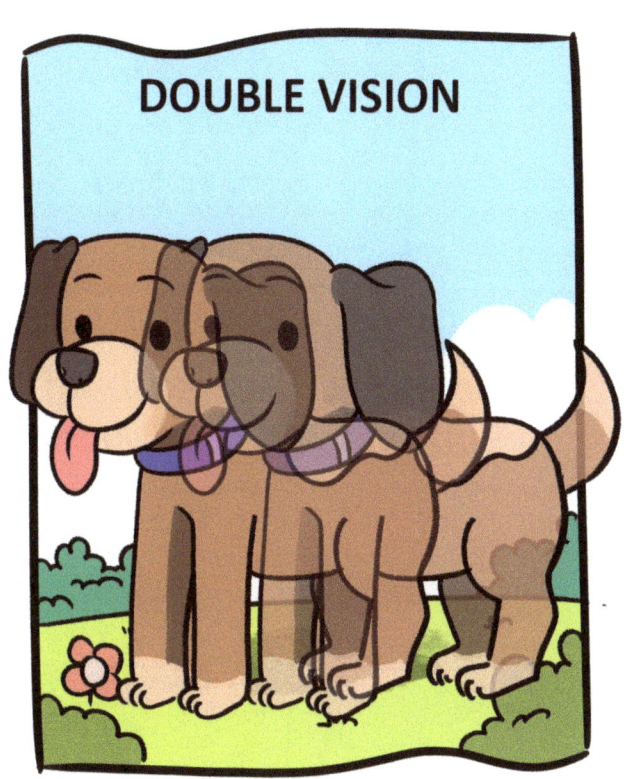

To help you see better, eye muscle surgery helps loosen tight muscles and tighten loose ones so both of your eyes can see things more clearly to help you learn and grow.

Here are some other eye surgeries for children.

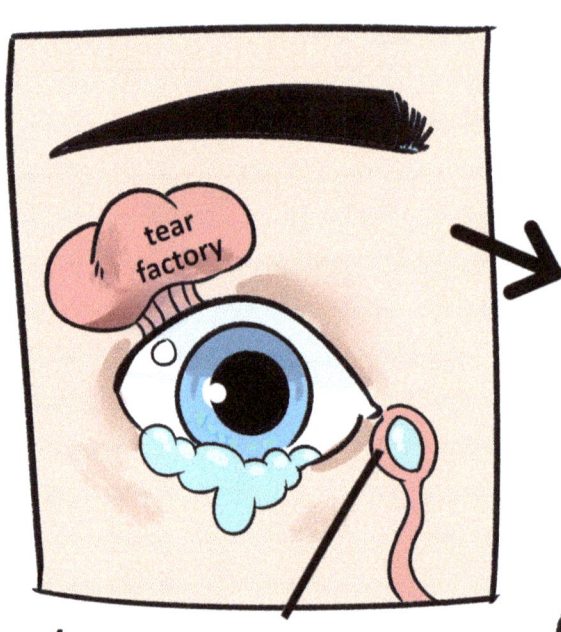

Tear duct (the tiny drain on the nasal corner of the eye) surgery - to open up blocked tear ducts

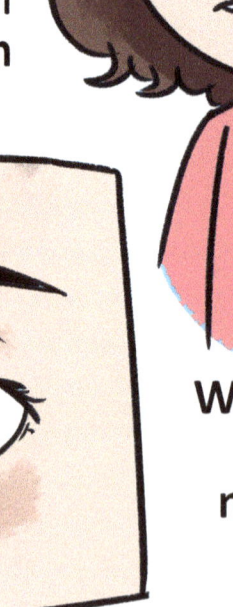

When the tear ducts are blocked, tears have nowhere to go, so the eyes get watery.

Eyelid surgery – to lift the eyelid so it doesn't cover the eye

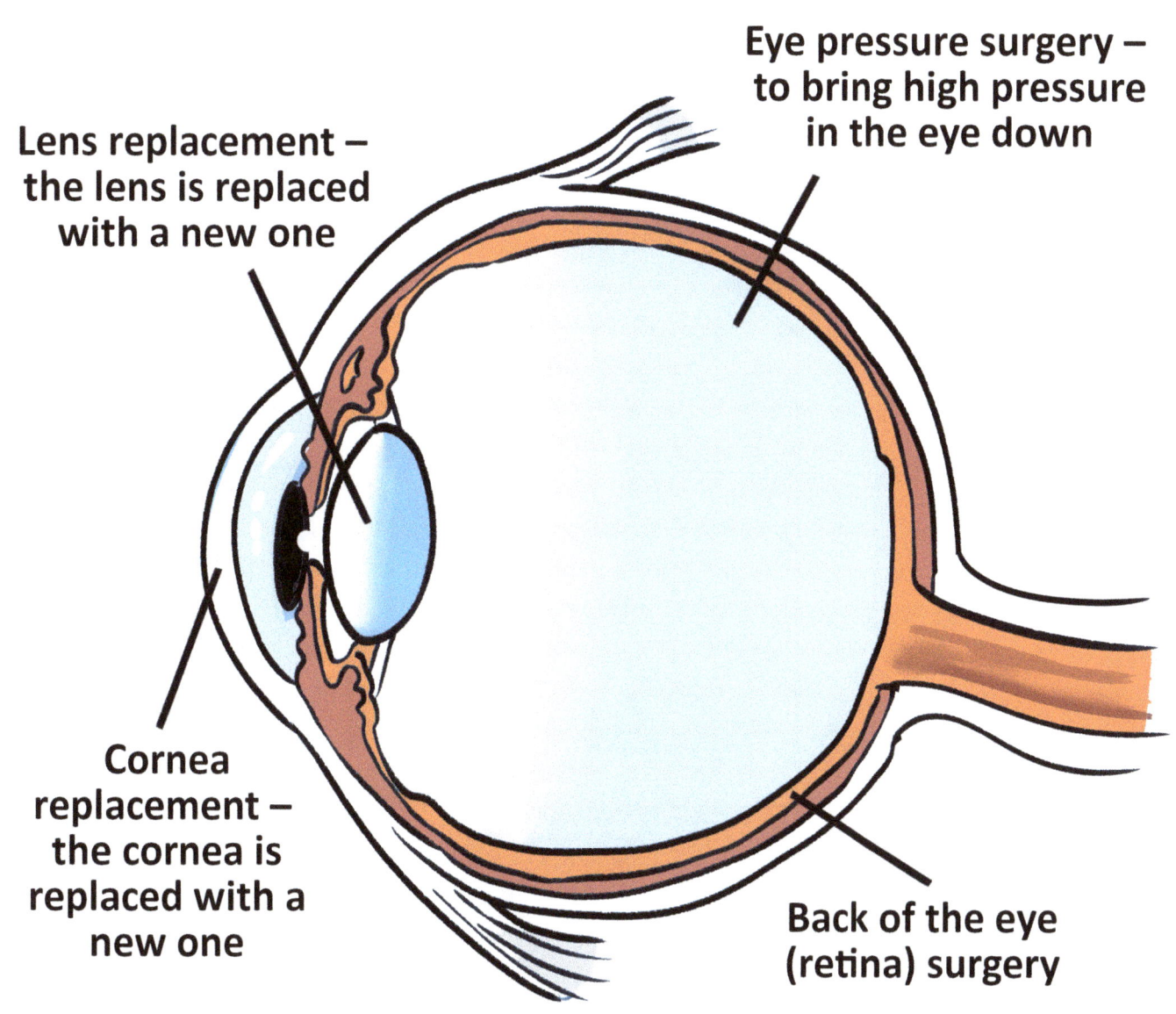

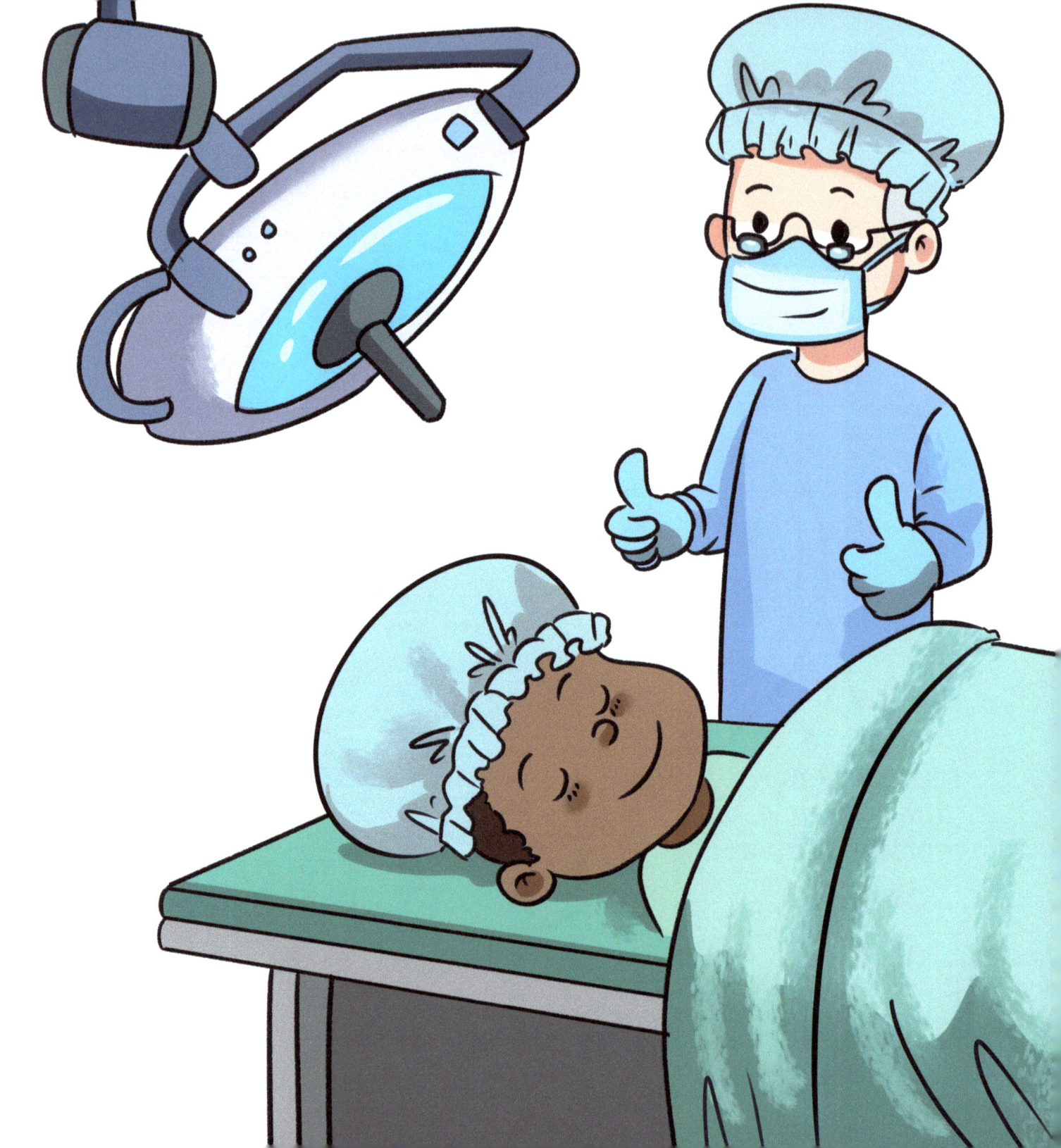

For your surgery, your friendly surgeon may use microscope glasses to help them see well and fix your eye.

Your doctors and nurses will keep you safe and comfortable.

You will be sleeping and dreaming away while the surgery is underway, and you won't feel a thing!

What do you want to dream about during your surgery?

Sweet dreams...

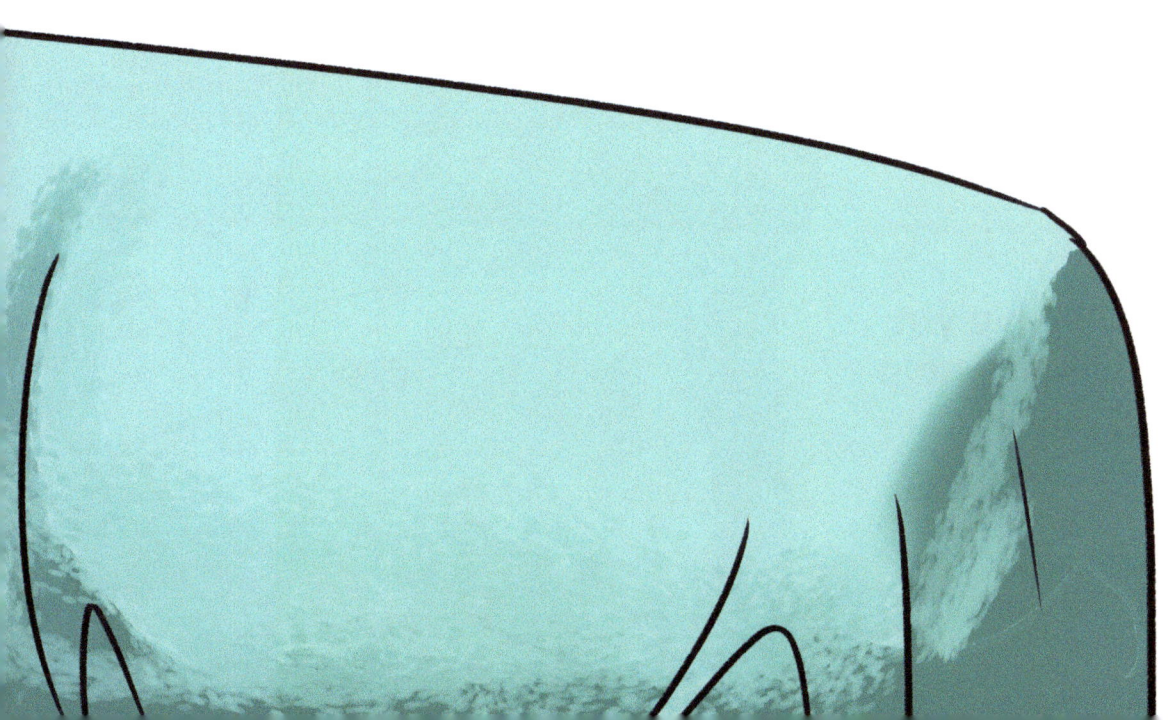

After your surgery, you will wake up in the hospital recovery room.

You may feel sleepy or sick to your stomach, and your eye may feel sore, scratchy, and uncomfortable.

Please remember not to touch or rub your eye.

Your nurse will give you special medicine to help you feel better.

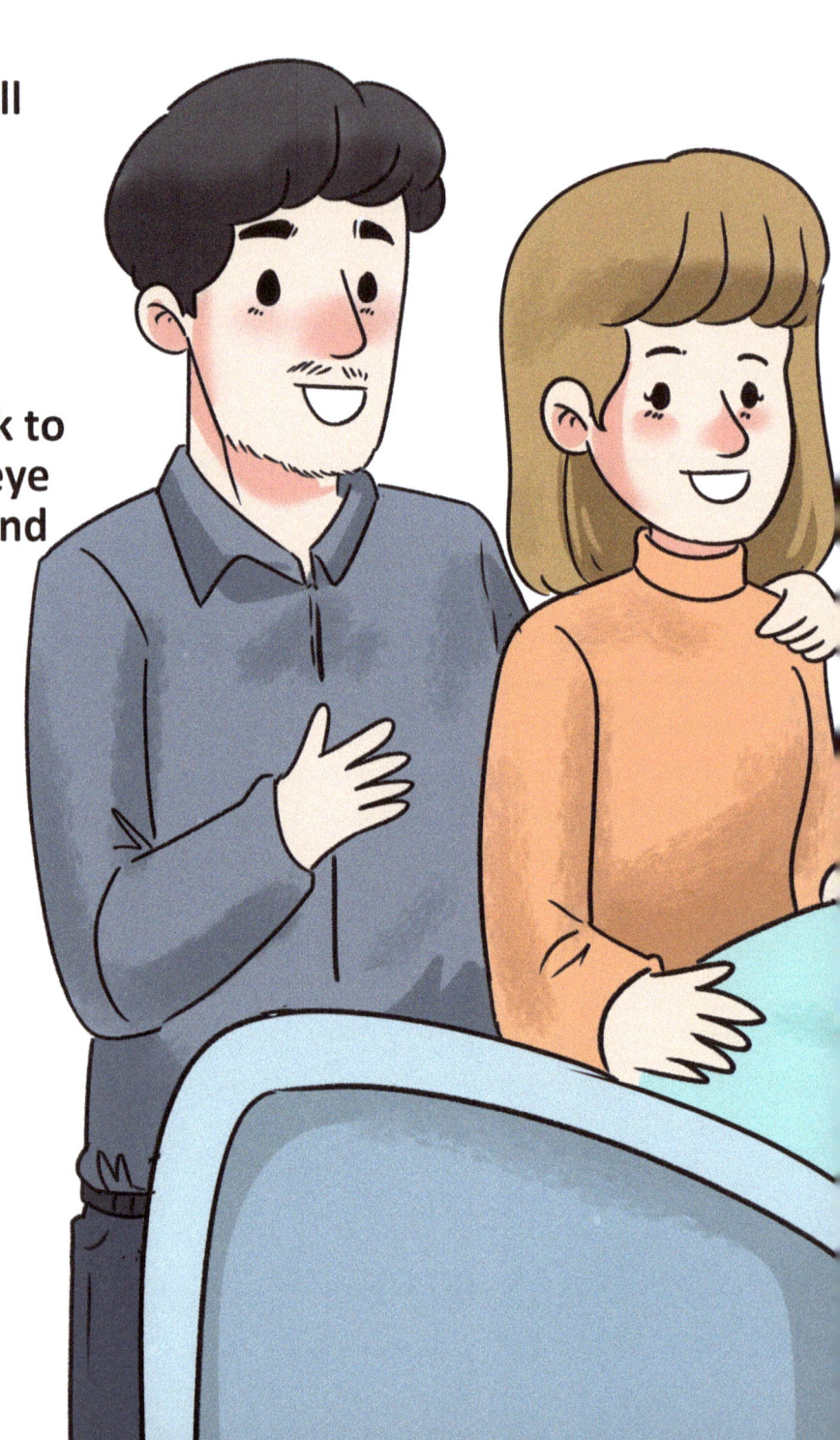

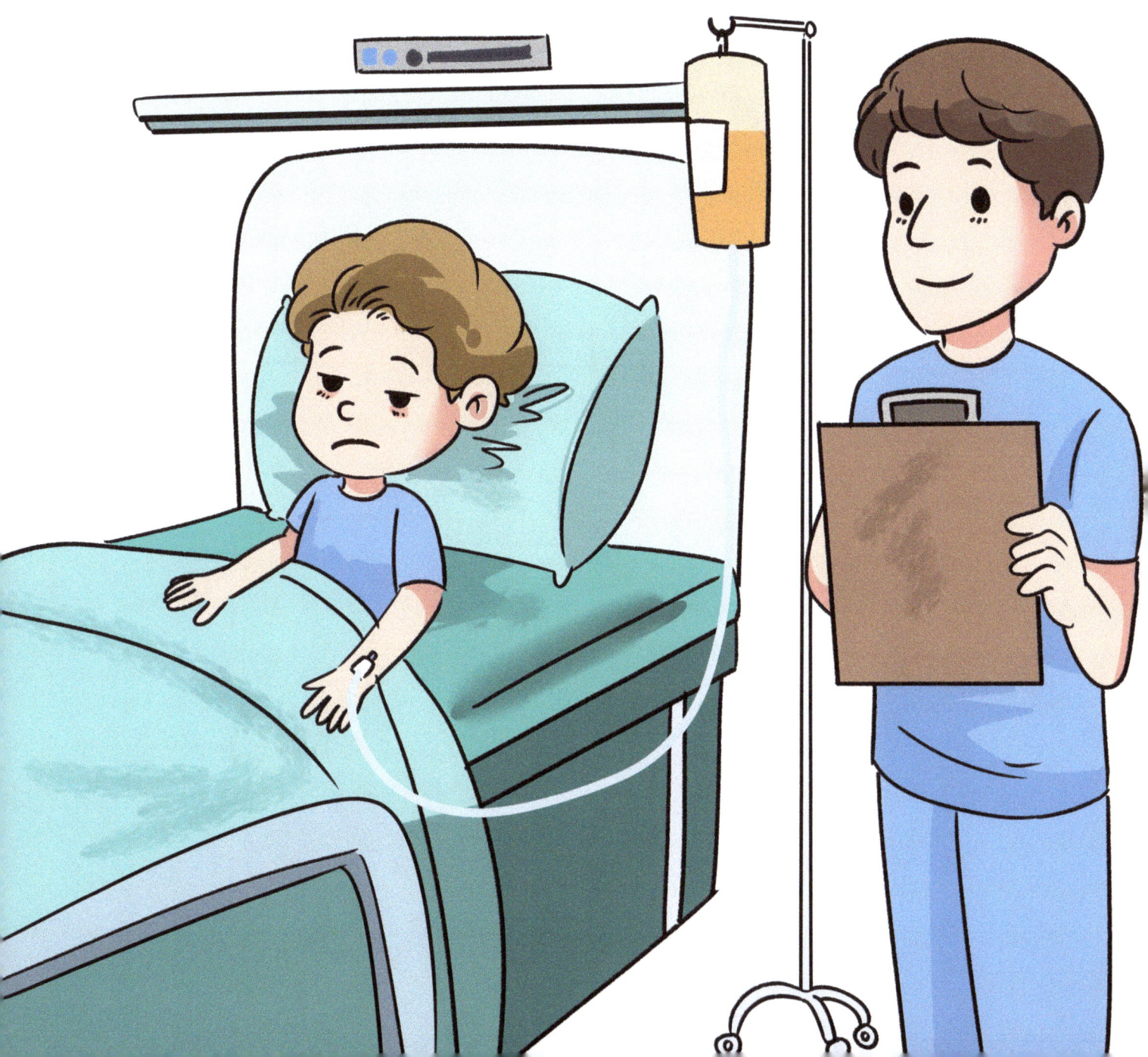

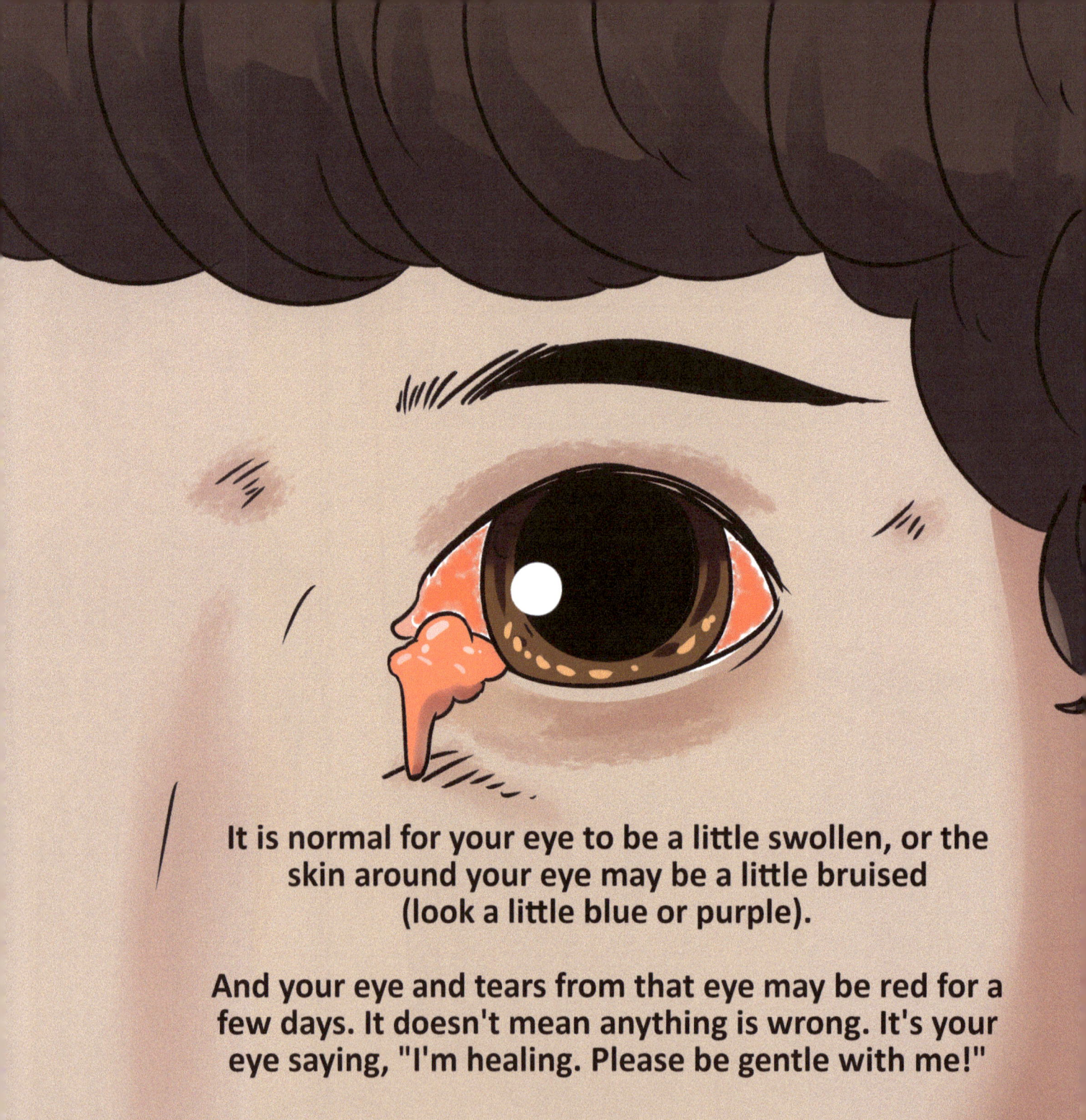

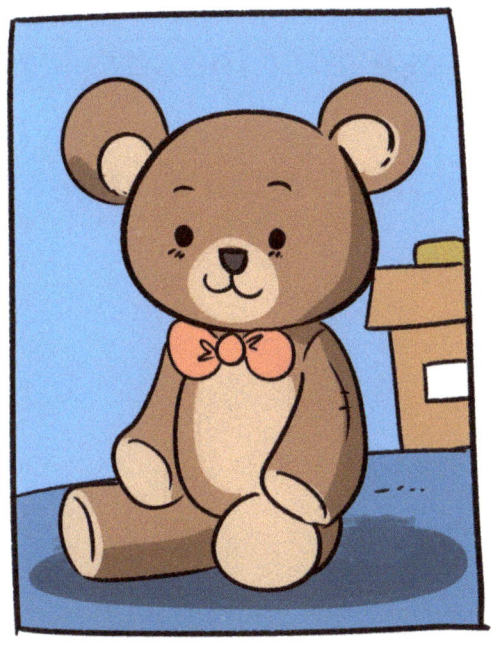

CLEAR

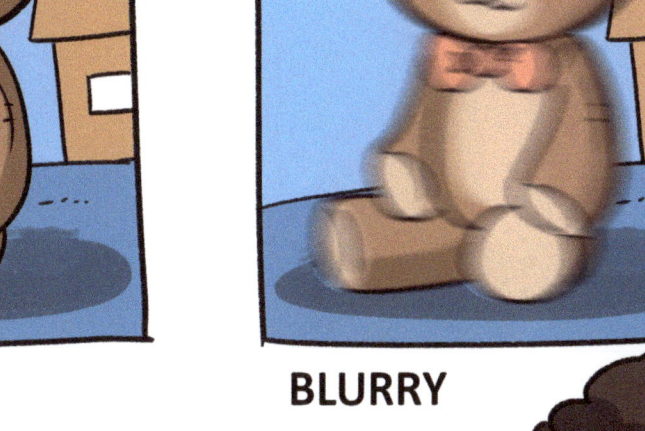

BLURRY

Your eye is getting better every day.

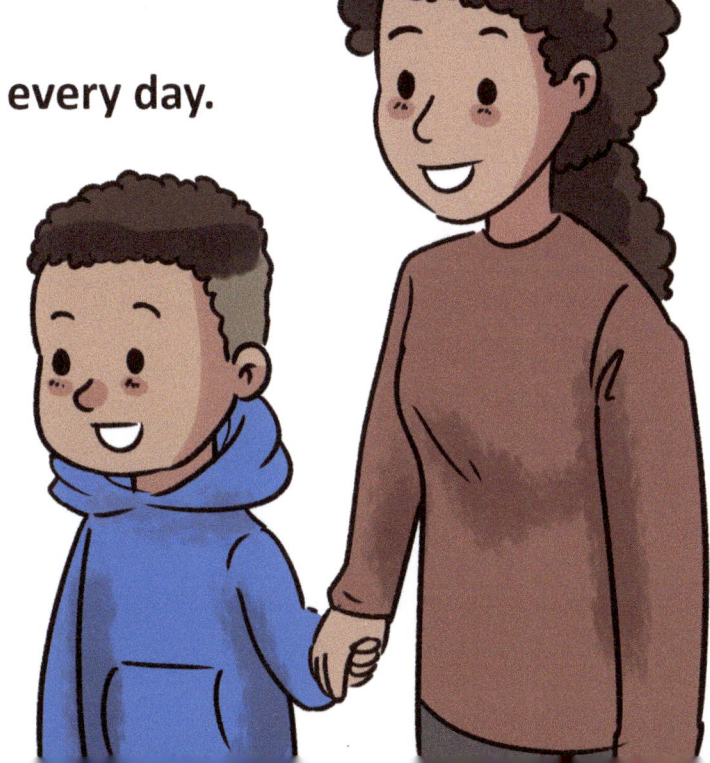

While your eye is healing, things might look blurry. So please ask a grown-up for help if you need to move around.

Depending on their eye surgery and needs, some children get a patch or shield over their eye after the surgery.

If you get an eye patch, it means your eye needs it to heal and get stronger. *Will you help your eye heal faster and get stronger?*

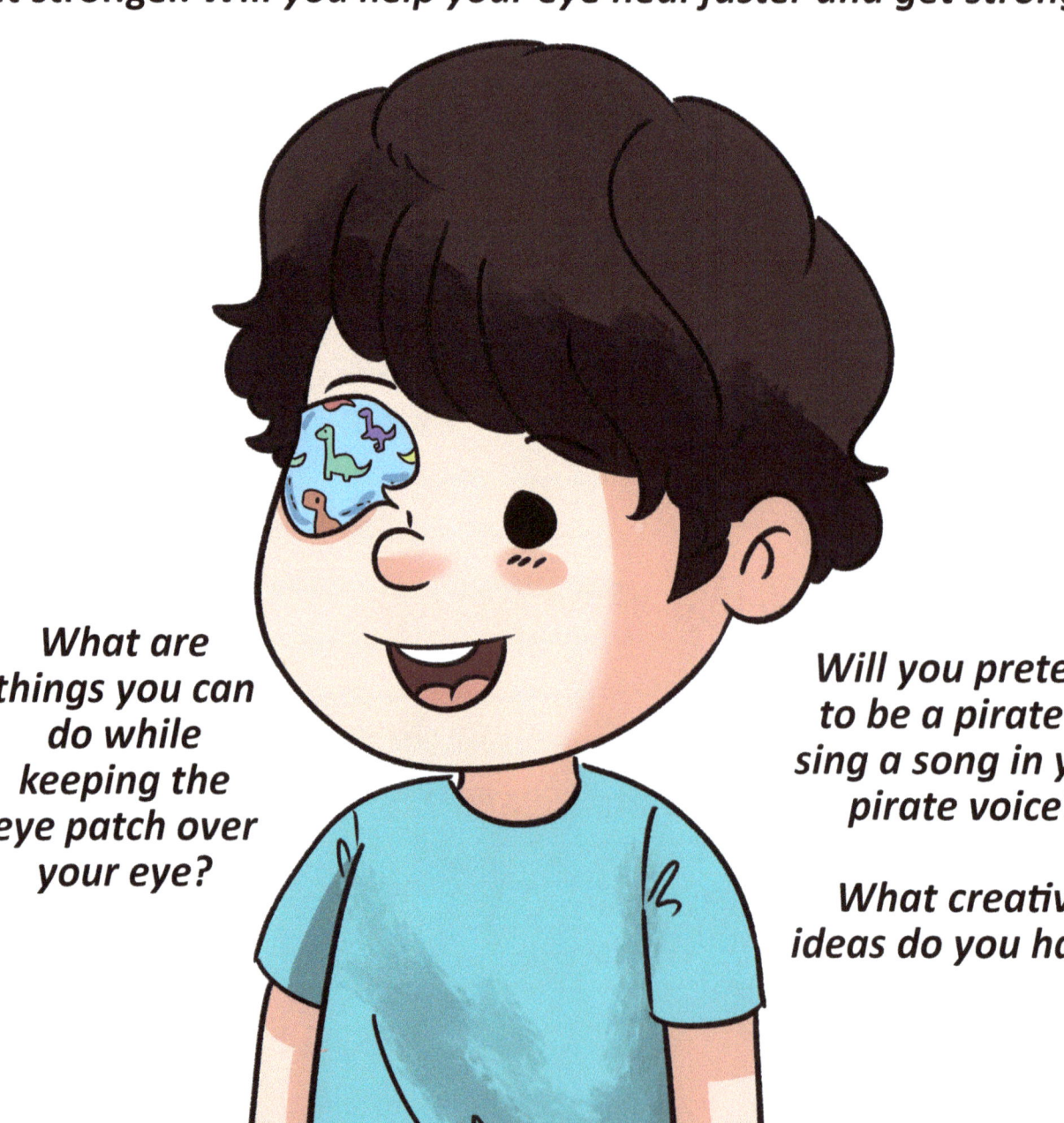

What are things you can do while keeping the eye patch over your eye?

Will you pretend to be a pirate or sing a song in your pirate voice?

What creative ideas do you have?

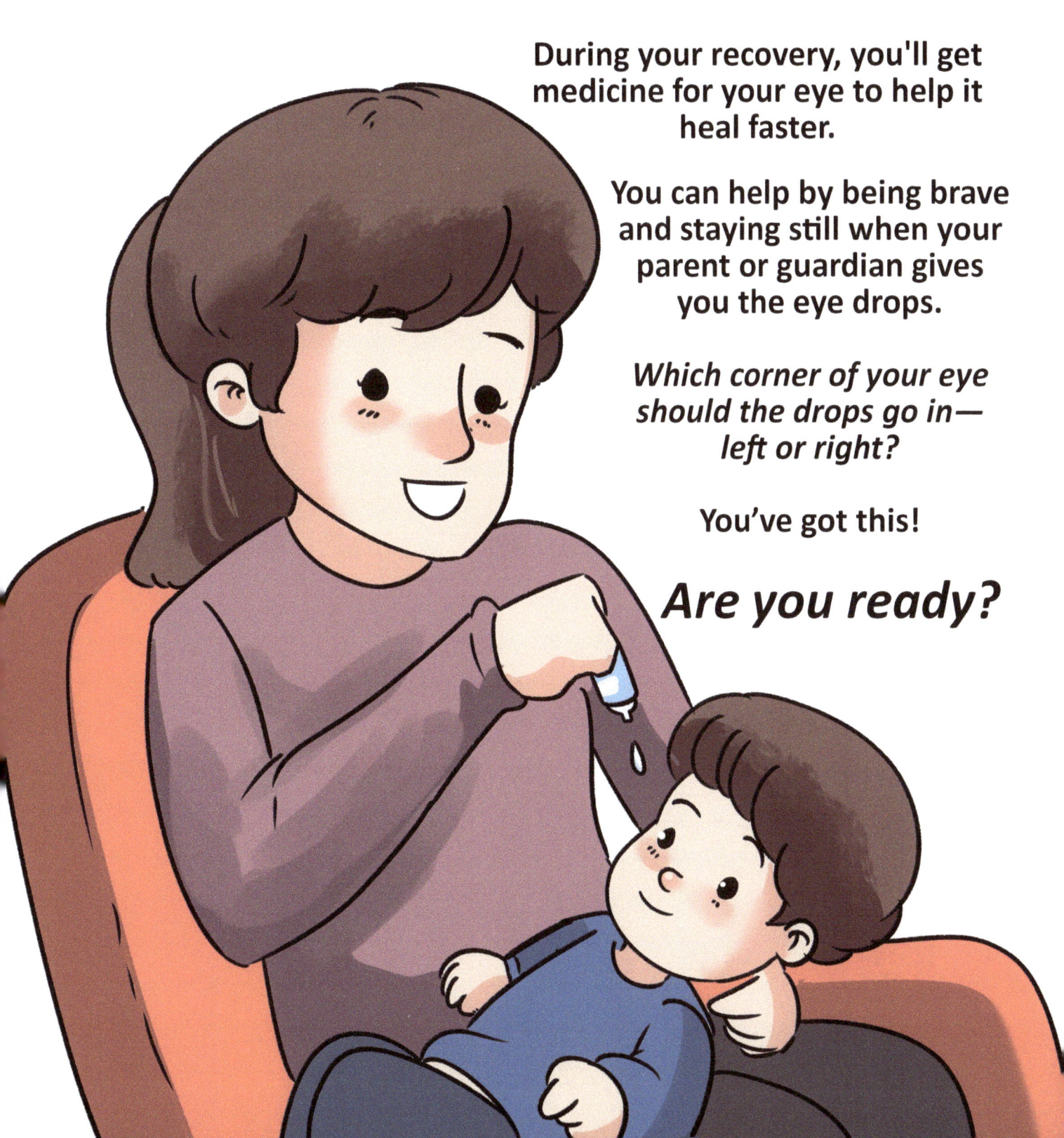

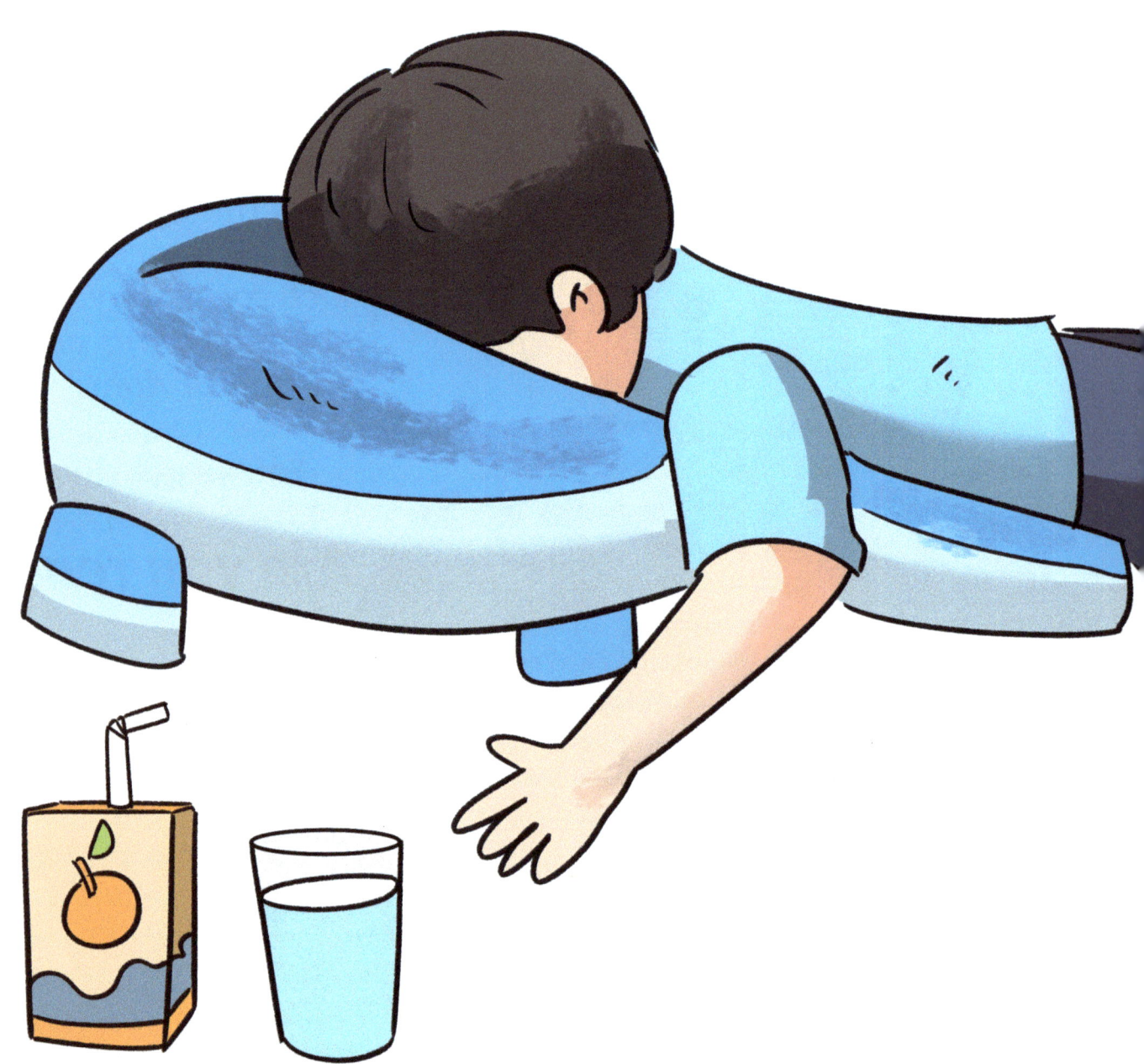

After retina surgery, some children need to rest and sleep on their belly, with their face down, for a while, using a special pillow to help their eye heal and get stronger.

If you have to sleep on your belly with your face down after your surgery, what are things you can do to make yourself more comfortable?

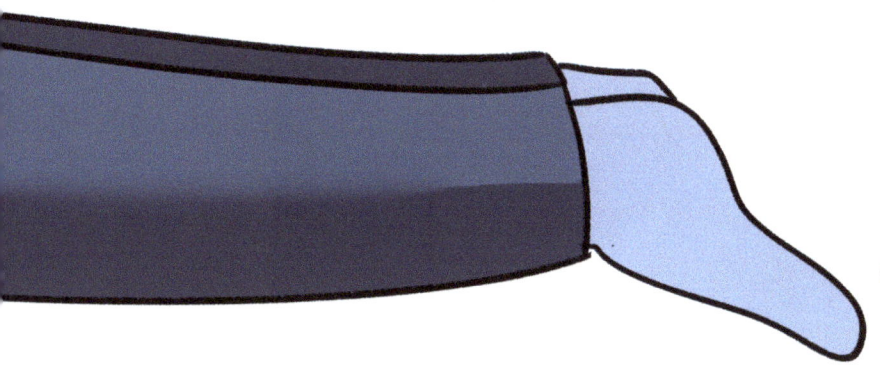

How about a pillow under your legs?

Or, listen to your favorite songs?

What ideas do you have?

You can do this!

When you're recovering from your surgery, please *relax* and take it easy!

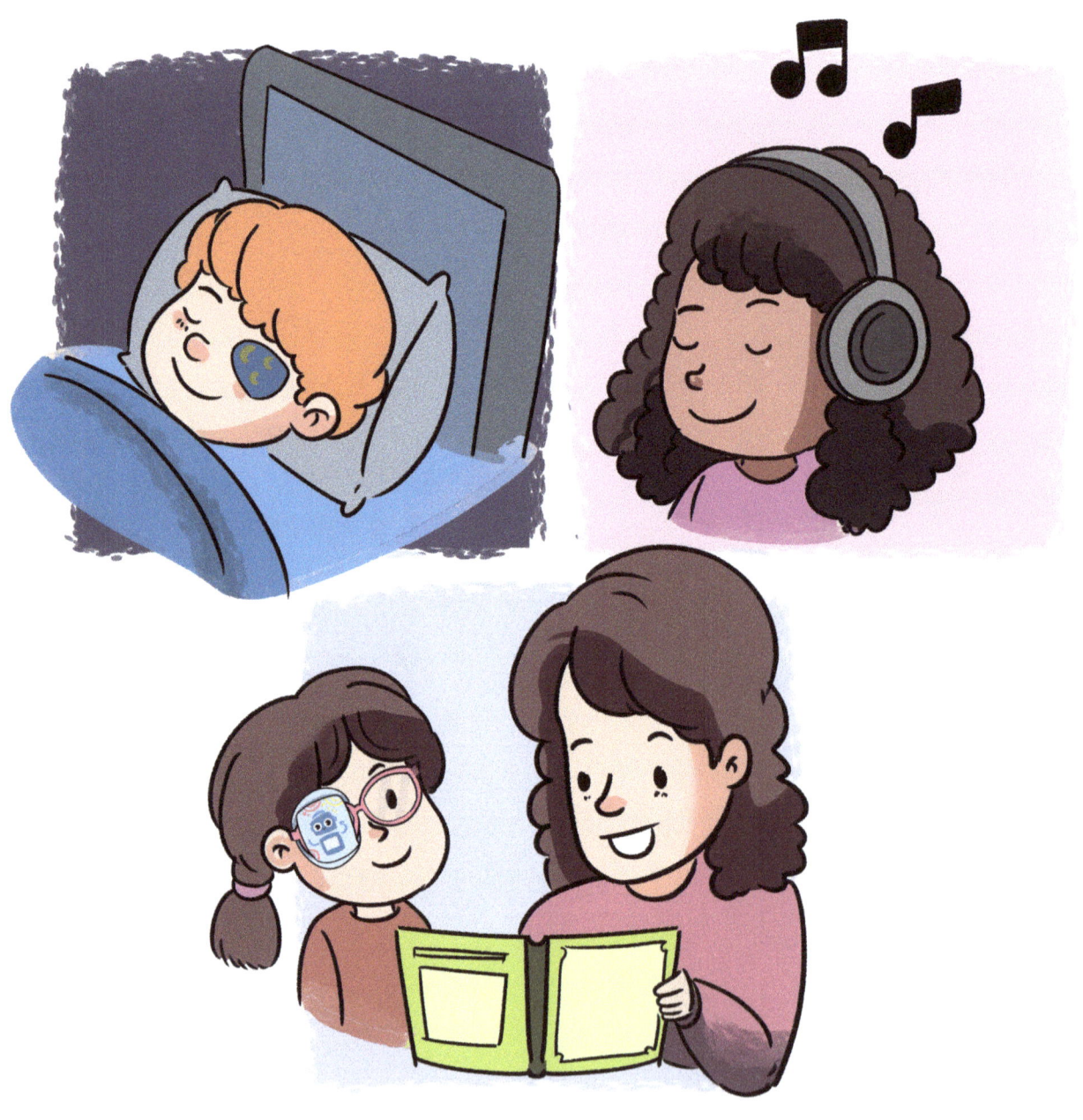

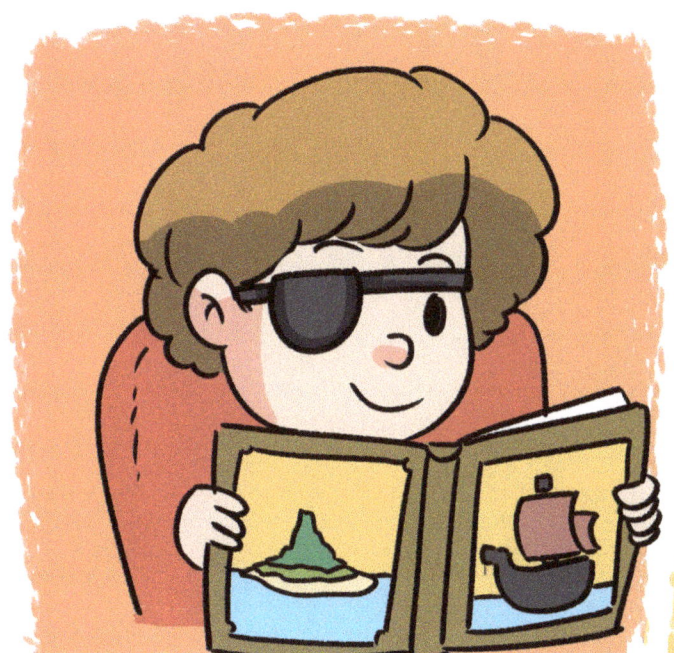

What do you plan to do?

- Rest with your favorite cozy blanket
- Listen to music
- Listen to stories
- Read a little
- Draw or color
- Watch a little bit of your favorite show

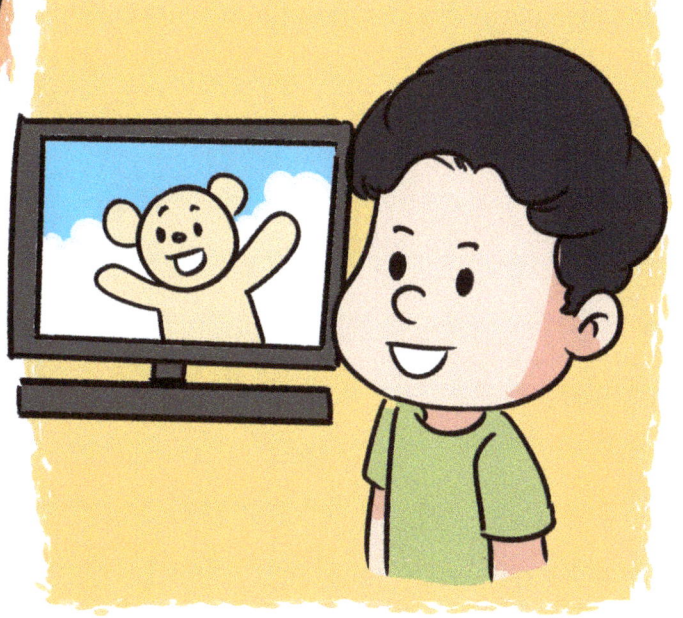

Say NO to activities that could hurt or put pressure on your eye, such as playing with balls, flying toys, contact sports, swimming, or running.

Please also remember to protect your eye from water, soap, and shampoo.

Don't worry; your doctor will tell your parent or guardian how to take care of your eye while it's healing.

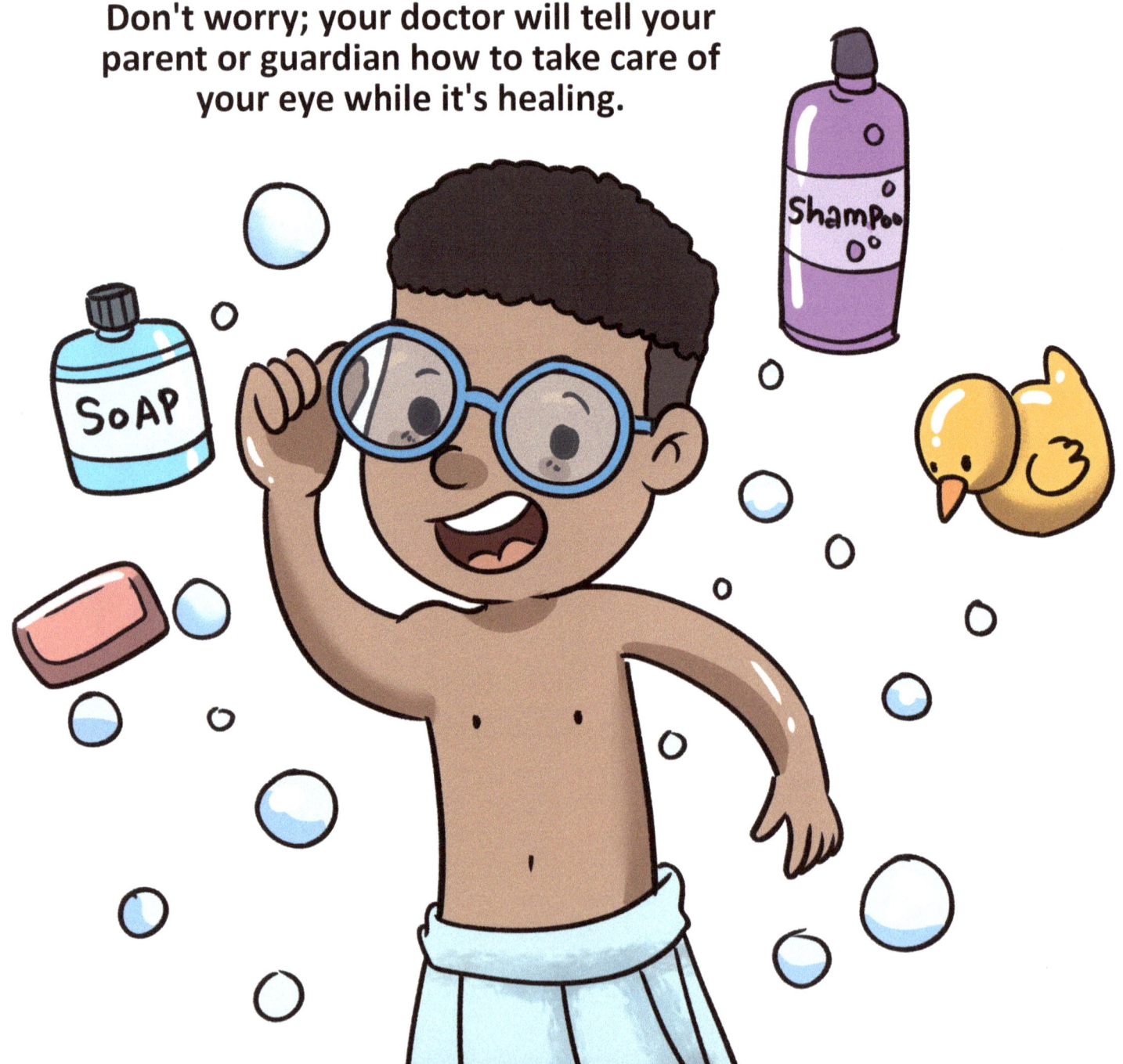

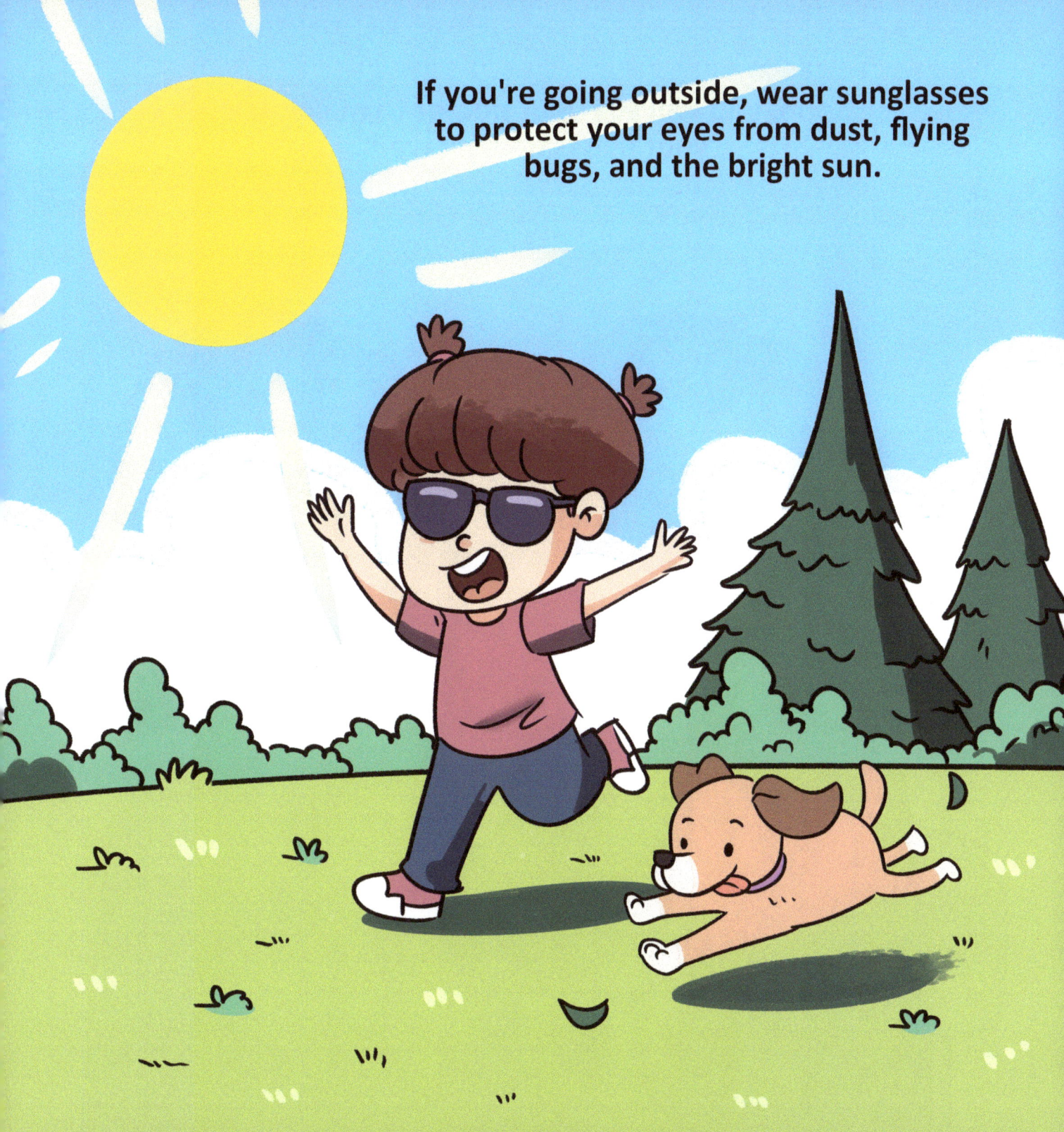

Soon, you will see your doctor to make sure your eye is healing well.

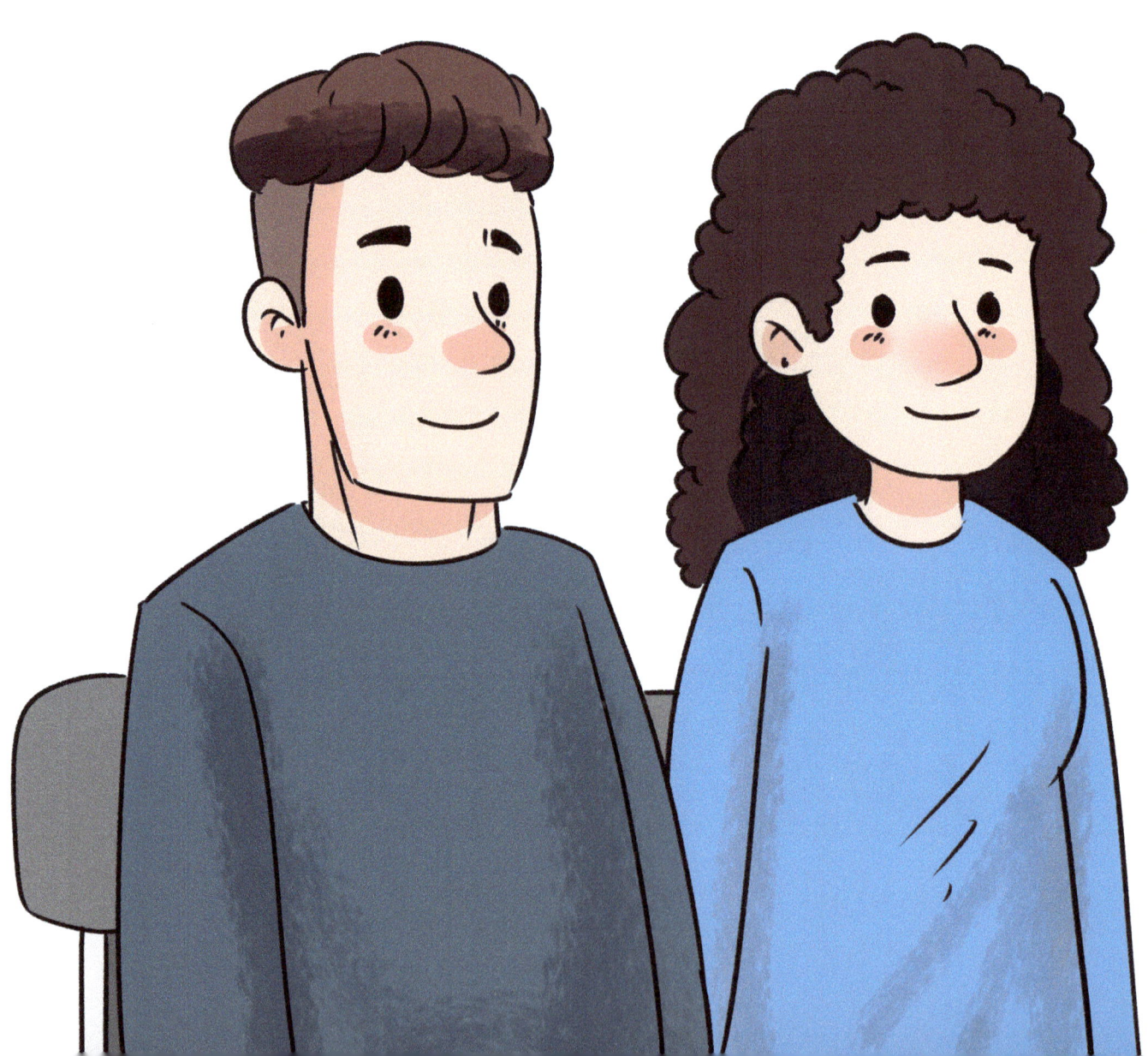

If you have questions about your eye, feel free to ask your doctor. Please write your questions below.

_____

_____

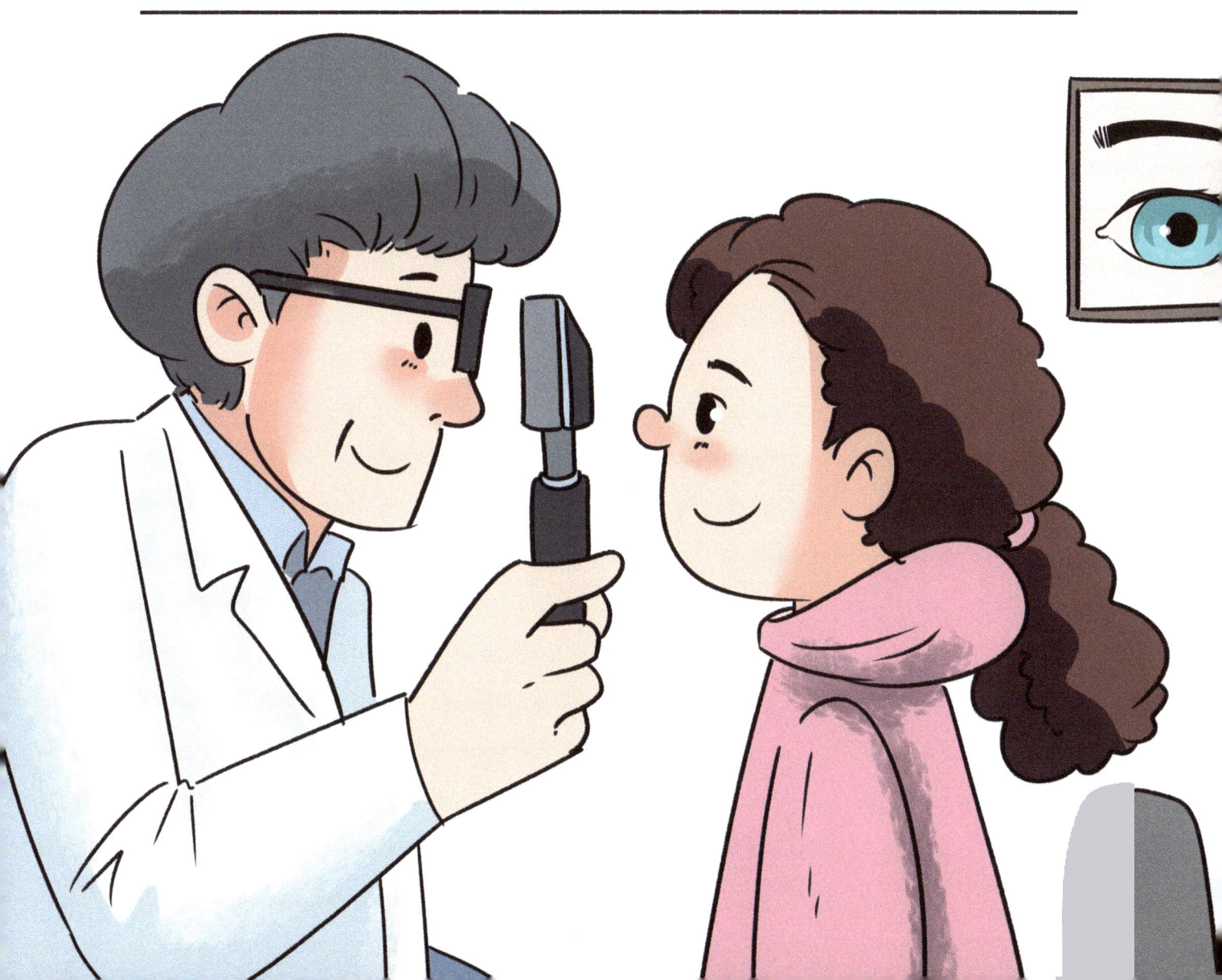

What will you do after your eye surgery?

A party? A celebration?

What's your favorite way to celebrate?

Draw or write your party plan below.

Speedy recovery!

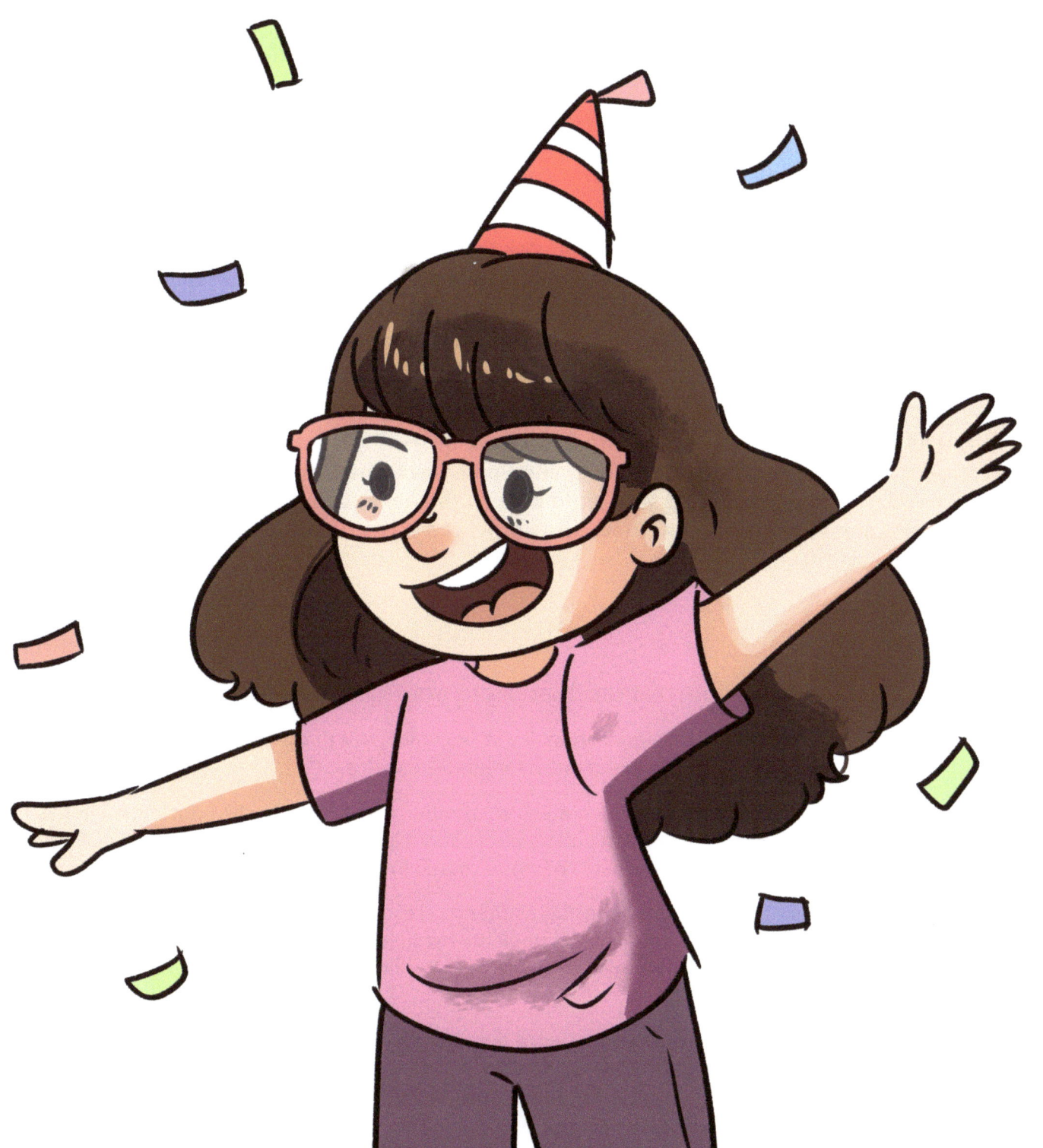

Notes for Parent/Guardian

- Placement of the intravenous (IV) catheter in this young age group is typically done *after* your child is asleep in the operating room.

- After the surgery, it is common for children to feel confused, disoriented, or irritable, and they may cry, sob, kick, scream, or thrash around.
It normally takes about one hour for the anesthesia to wear off.

- Applying eye drops: Keep the tip of the eye drop bottle clean. It may be easier to place the drops in the corner of your child's eye and then ask them to blink a few times to help spread the medicine. Before leaving the hospital, you can ask the medical staff for a small bottle of balanced salt solution (BSS) so your child can practice on a stuffed animal to help them feel more confident. BSS is also available over the counter at most local pharmacies.

- Post-surgery instructions/restrictions:
Your child's doctor should give you specific instructions on (1) what your child can and cannot do during the recovery period, (2) the duration of the post-surgical restrictions, and (3) any post-surgical follow-ups. Additionally, (4) they should instruct what to watch out for and when it is necessary for you to bring your child back to the hospital in case of an emergency.
If they forget, please kindly remind them and obtain these instructions/restrictions before leaving the hospital.

Disclaimer

Please note that the illustrations are not drawn to scale.

This book is written for informational, educational, and personal growth purposes and should not be used as a substitute for medical advice.

Please consult your child's doctor if they need medical attention and to ensure the information in this book pertains to your child's medical condition and needs. I cannot guarantee what your child experiences is exactly what is being discussed in this book.

The author and the publisher are not responsible, either directly or indirectly, for any damages, monetary losses, or reparations due to information in this book. By reading this book, the readers agree not to hold the author and the publisher responsible for any losses as a result of any errors, inaccuracies, or omissions in this book.

Please keep in mind that your child's experience depends on the location, the facility, their medical condition, and the healthcare team. Please use this book in conjunction with your child's doctor's advice.
Thank you.

Did this picture book help your child in some way?
If so, I would love to hear about it!

www.amazon.com/gp/product-review/B0F4PC429M

For other book titles, please visit:

www.fzwbooks.com

Connect with the author

email: books@fzwbooks.com
facebook/instagram: @FZWbooks

About the Author

Dr. Fei Zheng-Ward is a clinical anesthesiologist who understands the apprehension patients (both adults and children) may have surrounding their upcoming surgery. Her goal in her medical books is to bring useful information to patients so they have a better understanding and appreciation of what happens leading up to, during, and after surgery. She wants readers to be more empowered to make informed decisions and to feel more at ease with their surgery.

As a practicing physician, she takes pride in being respected for her attention to detail, commitment to providing compassionate and personalized patient care, and strong presence in patient advocacy in the perioperative period for each of her patients. She understands the importance of physical and emotional well-being and advocates for patient autonomy.

Her other children's books aim to bring laughter into your family, encourage children to be more helpful at home, and inspire a love of reading.

She is an award-winning author for her book titled ***What to Expect and How to Prepare for Your Surgery***.

More about Dr. Fei Zheng-Ward:

- Board Certified Anesthesiologist

- Anesthesiology Residency Training at The Johns Hopkins Hospital in Baltimore, MD

- Master in Public Health (MPH) degree from Dartmouth Medical School in Hanover, NH

Books by the author

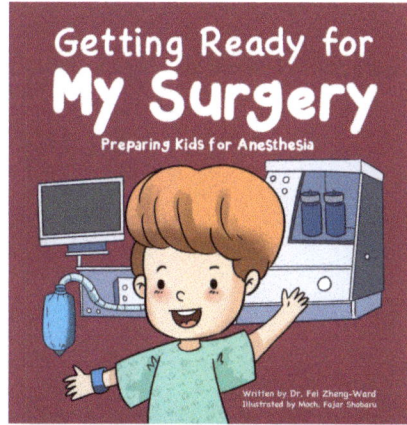
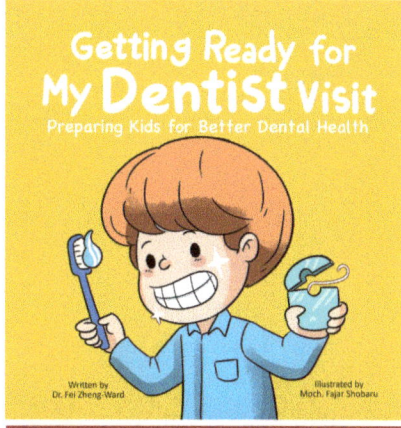
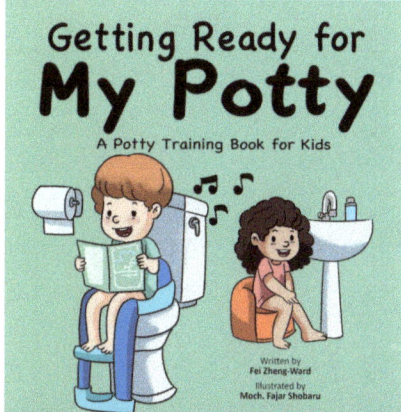
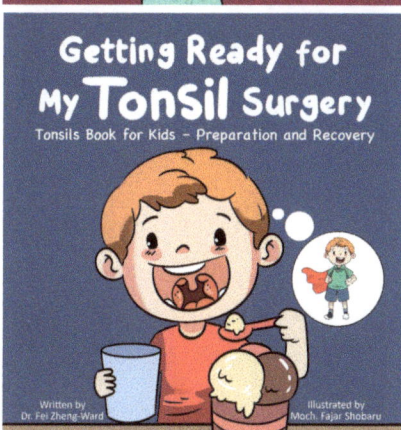
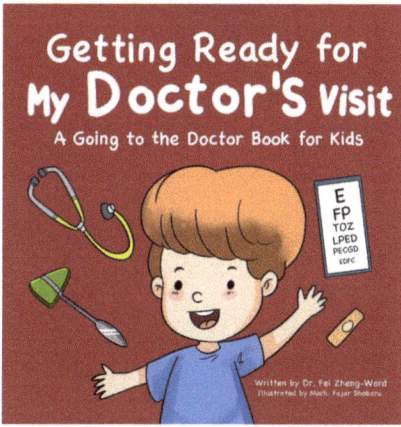
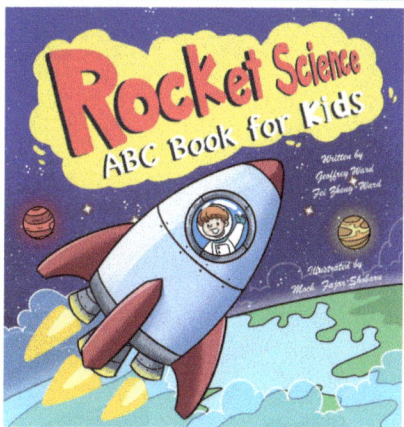
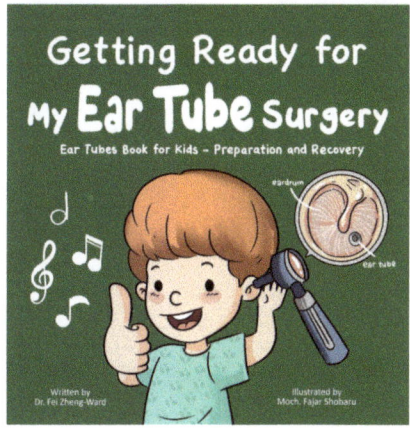
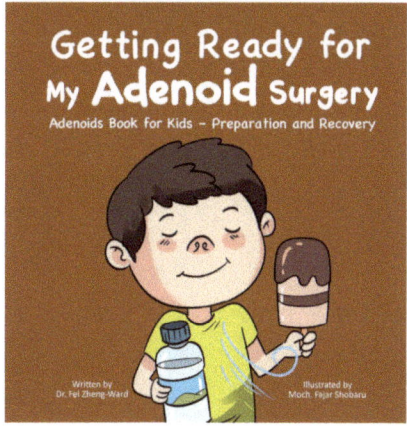
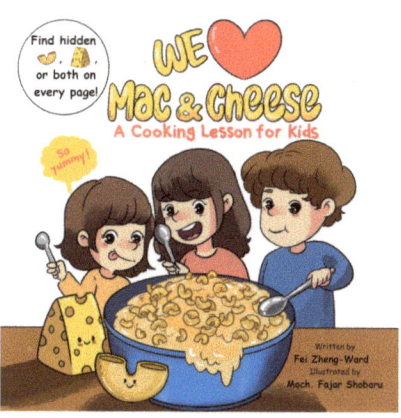

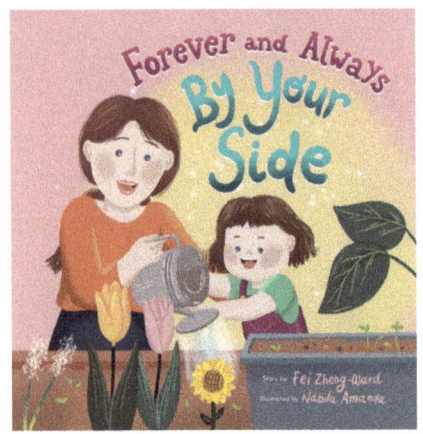
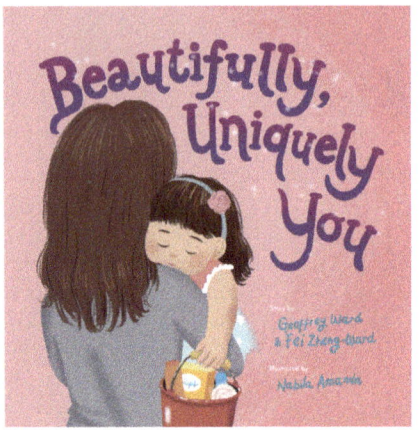
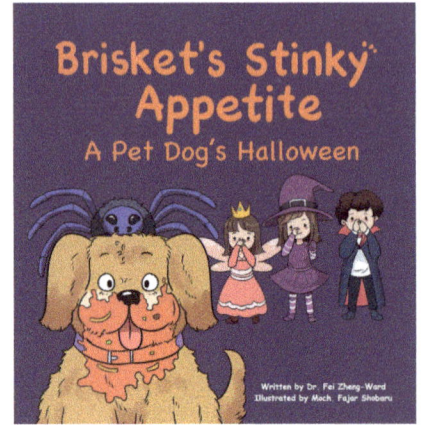
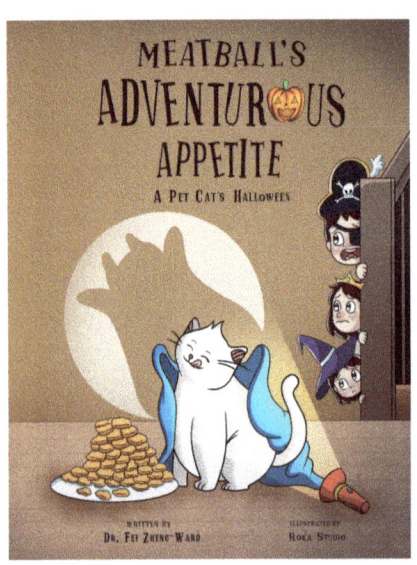
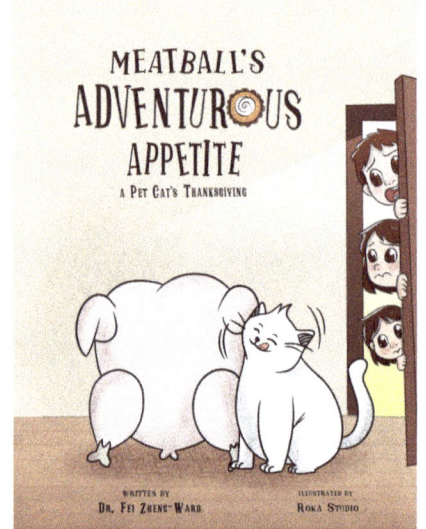
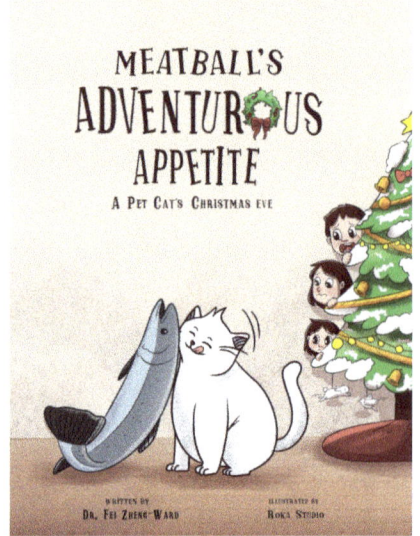
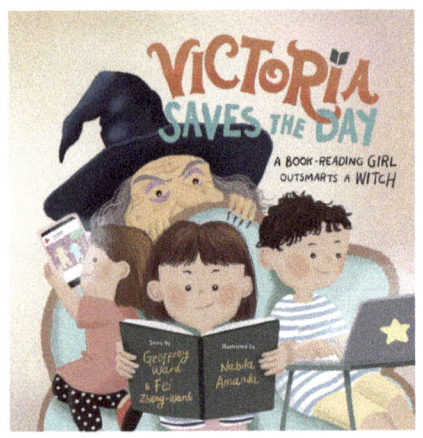
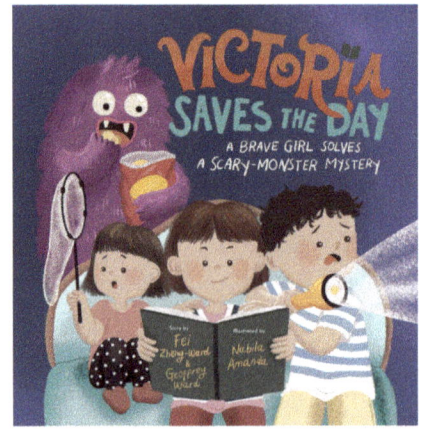
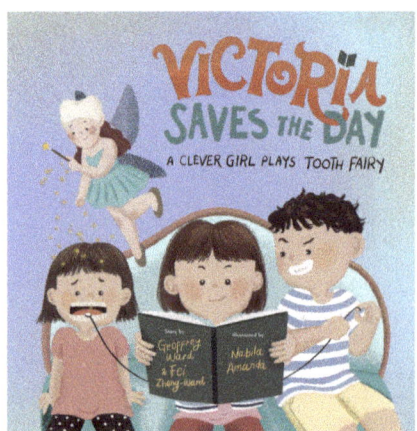

www.ingramcontent.com/pod-product-compliance
Lightning Source LLC
Chambersburg PA
CBHW040001040426
42337CB00032B/5185